Knee Ligament Injuries

Roberto Rossi • Fabrizio Margheritini
Editors

Knee Ligament Injuries

Extraarticular Surgical Techniques

Springer

Editors
Roberto Rossi
Mauriziano "Umberto I" Hospital
Turin
Italy

Fabrizio Margheritini
University of Rome "Foro Italico"
Rome
Italy

ISBN 978-88-470-5874-3 ISBN 978-88-470-5513-1 (eBook)
DOI 10.1007/978-88-470-5513-1
Springer Milan Heidelberg New York Dordrecht London

Printed on acid-free paper

Springer is part of Springer Science+Business Media (www.springer.com)

Preface

Extra-articular reconstruction has been employed over the past century to address anterior cruciate ligament (ACL) deficiency, but the technique has not gained favor owing primarily to residual instability and secondarily to the development of degenerative changes in the lateral and medial compartments of the knee. As a consequence, intra-articular arthroscopic reconstruction has become the technique of choice. However, we know from several clinical and biomechanical studies that intra-articular reconstruction, despite the introduction of so-called anatomical reconstruction, does not completely restore normal knee kinematics. Therefore some authors have recommended extra-articular reconstruction in conjunction with an intra-articular technique.

This book provides in-depth descriptions of the extra-articular surgical techniques that may be employed when performing ligament reconstruction in patients with injuries involving the posterolateral and posteromedial corners of the knee. It is intended as a practical, "how to" manual that will be of value for both the trainee and the more experienced surgeon. Many of the techniques relate to the central pivot of the knee, i.e., the anterior and posterior cruciate ligaments. For each technique, indications, presurgical planning, postsurgical follow-up, and complications are discussed in addition to the surgical details. Numerous tips and pearls are provided and the techniques are clearly depicted in informative high-quality illustrations.

Rome, Italy — Fabrizio Margheritini
Turin, Italy — Roberto Rossi

Acknowledgments

Writing this book would not have been possible without the help of many people, to whom we would like to express our gratitude.

First of all, we thank the Magellan Society, an International Society that brings together as members the Traveling Fellows and the guiding Godparents of different Sports Medicine societies across the world. Among the members of this society we found the contributors to this book, who we thank for sharing their expertise and for presenting what we believe to be the most complete and up-to-date guidance on the diagnosis and treatment of peripheral instability. The value of this book lies only in the knowledge of these authors.

Then we would like to thank our families for allowing us to spend time over this project without feeling too much guilt.

We also wish to thank the staff at Springer for overseeing the entire publication process until the release of the book.

Finally, we would like to thank Dr. John A. Feagin and Dr. Werner Muller, whose work inspired the idea of writing this book.

Contents

What Is New in Knee Surgery?

1

Matthew J. Boyle and Dean C. Taylor

As is often said, what was once old is now new again. In recent years, the traditional orthopedic principle of restoration of anatomy has experienced a renaissance within the field of extra-articular knee reconstruction. Knee surgeons have moved again toward more anatomic restoration, while continuing to develop extra-articular augmentation procedures to protect these anatomic reconstructions.

For anterior cruciate ligament (ACL) injuries, extra-articular knee reconstruction initially became popular in the late 1960s, when the focus of treating patients with ACL injury began to move from anatomic primary repair to extra-articular reconstructions using local structures. Early techniques such as the Slocum and Larson [1], Losee et al. [2], Ellison [3], and Andrews and Sanders [4] procedures were developed in an attempt to control rotational instability of the knee utilizing extra-articular biomechanics. With advancing anatomic and biomechanical understanding and with technological development, the treatment of ACL injury has now evolved into an anatomic intra-articular reconstruction; however, these early extra-articular techniques remain useful as conjunct procedures in the dramatically unstable or revision reconstructive knee [5].

As has been the case for ACL injuries, there also has been a renewed emphasis on anatomic reconstruction procedures for other knee ligament injuries. Interesting recent developments in the field of extra-articular knee reconstruction include advances in the anatomic management of patellofemoral instability, posterolateral corner injury, medial collateral ligament injury, and pediatric ACL injury and in the understanding of allograft and platelet-rich plasma use.

M.J. Boyle (✉) • D.C. Taylor
Department of Orthopaedic Surgery, Duke University,
280 Frank Bassett Drive, Durham, NC 27710, USA
e-mail: matthew.j.boyle@dm.duke.edu; dean.taylor@duke.edu

R. Rossi, F. Margheritini (eds.), *Knee Ligament Injuries*,
DOI 10.1007/978-88-470-5513-1_1, © Springer Verlag Italia 2014

1.1 Patellofemoral Instability

Medial patellofemoral ligament (MPFL) reconstruction has become a popular surgical option in the management of patellofemoral instability in select patients. Recently, Fulkerson and Edgar have suggested that the MPFL reconstruction may be anatomically incorrect [6]. Through detailed anatomic dissections of the deep medial knee retinaculum, Fulkerson and Edgar have demonstrated a consistent prominent structure extending from the distal deep quadriceps tendon to the adductor tubercle region, forming a distinct medial quadriceps tendon-femoral ligament (MQTFL). In their published series, reconstruction of this anatomic structure yielded consistent medial stabilization of the patellofemoral joint without drilling into the patella in 17 patients with recurrent patella instability with greater than 12 months follow-up [6]. Further research is required to investigate the anatomic and functional importance of the MQTFL.

1.2 Posterolateral Corner Injury

Although posterolateral corner (PLC) injuries may occur in conjunction with up to 7.5 % of ACL injuries [7], this combined injury pattern is still often missed. Failure of recognition and appropriate treatment of PLC injury places increased stress on ACL reconstructions and may predispose patients to early graft failure. Anatomic extra-articular restoration of injured PLC structures will likely protect anatomic ACL reconstruction and optimize functional outcome in patients presenting with this combined injury. Kim et al. recently demonstrated that within a population of 425 patients, 32 patients who presented with combined PLC and ACL injury and were managed with anatomic PLC and ACL reconstruction had significantly less anterior tibial translation and comparable functional outcome scores at 2 years postoperatively when compared to 393 patients with isolated ACL injury who were managed with ACL reconstruction alone [7]. Interestingly, in a recent cohort study, Yoon et al. found no objective or functional benefit to the addition of a popliteal tendon reconstruction in addition to an anatomic PLC reconstruction [8]. This illustrates the importance that knee surgeons remain focused on restoration of anatomy in order to achieve the best possible patient outcomes.

1.3 Medial Collateral Ligament Injury

Early medial collateral ligament (MCL) reconstruction involved nonanatomic sling-type procedures that frequently resulted in residual laxity, loss of knee motion, and disappointing patient outcomes. Over the past 10 years, a number of more anatomic procedures for MCL reconstruction have been developed, typically involving hamstring tendon graft with modern fixation devices to reconstruct the superficial MCL. These procedures have demonstrated improved results compared to early techniques; however, they fail to address the injured posteromedial structures in addition to the superficial MCL. Recently, LaPrade and Wijdicks, in conjunction with the University of Oslo, Norway, have undertaken detailed quantitative anatomic studies in addition to static and dynamic biomechanical studies in order to develop an anatomic medial knee reconstruction. LaPrade and Wijdicks' [9] technique consists of a reconstruction of the proximal and distal divisions of the superficial medial collateral ligament in addition to the posterior oblique ligament (POL) using two separate grafts. In a group of 28 patients with MCL insufficiency followed prospectively for an average of 18 months, LaPrade and Wijdicks found this anatomic technique to restore valgus, external rotation, and internal rotation stability and improve patient function [9]. Future medial knee reconstructions may benefit from the addition of POL reconstruction in order to truly restore patient anatomy and optimize postoperative function.

1.4 Pediatric Anterior Cruciate Ligament Injury

The optimal surgical technique in pediatric ACL reconstruction remains a source of much debate. Although recent literature suggests that transphyseal ACL reconstruction in Tanner stage 1 and 2 children can achieve satisfactory outcomes with low complication rates [10], the concern of growth disturbance continues to stimulate interest in potentially nonanatomic and extra-articular procedures in these young patients. Kennedy et al. recently undertook a biomechanical cadaveric study investigating three ACL reconstruction techniques that attempt to avoid disruption of the physis: the all-epiphyseal technique, the transtibial over-the-top technique, and the iliotibial band physeal-sparing technique [11]. All techniques restored some stability to the knee. The iliotibial band reconstruction best restored anteroposterior stability and rotational control, although it appeared to overconstrain the knee to rotational forces at some flexion angles.

1.5 Allograft Tissue

The use of allograft tissue in ligamentous knee reconstruction remains a topic of debate. The orthopedic community's understanding of allograft biomechanical properties continues to evolve. Allograft remains an excellent option in patients undergoing multiple ligament reconstruction in order to increase graft number, reduce donor site morbidity, and limit operative duration. Isolated MCL reconstruction also provides a suitable facet for allograft due to concern for donor site morbidity. Marx and Hetsroni recently published a technique to reconstruct the MCL using Achilles tendon allograft with encouraging results [12]. Despite these promising indications, the benefit of allograft reconstruction of isolated ACL injuries remains unclear. Spindler et al., in a study of 378 patients undergoing ACL reconstruction, recently demonstrated allograft use to be a significant predictor of poorer International Knee Documentation Committee and Knee Injury and Osteoarthritis Outcome Score outcomes at 6 years postoperatively [13].

1.6 Platelet-Rich Plasma

Platelet-rich plasma (PRP) therapy has been introduced to orthopedic surgery with the aim of enhancing tissue healing by increasing the concentration of growth factors and thereby moderating the inflammatory response, increasing cell migration, and stimulating angiogenesis. While basic science and laboratory studies have suggested that PRP therapy shows promise in a number of orthopedic subspecialties, the clinical significance of this therapy remains unclear. The majority of PRP research in knee ligamentous surgery has focused on ACL reconstruction. Although the basic science results have been encouraging, there unfortunately have only been two recent randomized trials investigating the effect of PRP on clinical outcomes. Mirzatolooei et al., in a randomized controlled trial of 50 patients undergoing ACL reconstruction using hamstring autograft, demonstrated no significant difference in clinical outcomes of bone tunnel widening between patients who had PRP introduced into tibial and femoral bone tunnels perioperatively and patients who did not [14]. Cervellin et al., in a randomized controlled trial of 40 patients undergoing ACL reconstruction with bone-patellar tendon-bone autograft, identified a small improvement in Victorian Institute Sport Assessment scale but no difference in visual analog pain scale or donor site bony healing in patients who had PRP gel applied to patellar and tibial bone harvest sites compared to patients who did not receive PRP gel [15]. Clinical studies have yet to convincingly support the use of platelet-rich plasma in knee ligamentous reconstruction.

Conclusion

Extra-articular knee reconstruction has evolved to a state where surgeons have seen improved results when advances in biological and anatomic understanding are applied to surgical techniques. This chapter has outlined many of the recent advances that have improved knee surgery outcomes.

The Magellan Orthopaedic Society has contributed significantly to the advancement of knee surgery through international collaboration of some of the world's most exceptional orthopedic sports medicine specialists. The talented Magellan members' chapters in this book will dive deeply into the internationally derived knowledge and provide thoughtful and creative solutions to challenging knee injuries.

References

1. Slocum DB, Larson RL (1968) Pes anserinus transplantation. A surgical procedure for control of rotatory instability of the knee. J Bone Joint Surg Am 50:211–225
2. Losee RE, Johnson TR, Southwick WO (1978) Anterior subluxation of the lateral tibial plateau. A diagnostic test and operative repair. J Bone Joint Surg Am 60:1015–1030
3. Ellison AE (1979) Distal iliotibial band transfer for anterolateral rotatory instability of the knee. J Bone Joint Surg Am 61:330–337

4. Andrews JR, Sanders R (1983) A "mini-reconstruction" technique in treating anterolateral rotatory instability (ALRI). Clin Orthop Relat Res 172:93–96
5. Trojani C, Beaufils P, Burdin G, Bussière C, Chassaing V, Djian P, Dubrana F, Ehkirch FP, Franceschi JP, Hulet C, Jouve F, Potel JF, Sbihi A, Neyret P, Colombet P (2012) Revision ACL reconstruction: influence of a lateral tenodesis. Knee Surg Sports Traumatol Arthrosc 20:1565–1570
6. Fulkerson JP, Edgar C (2013) Medial quadriceps tendon–femoral ligament: surgical anatomy and reconstruction technique to prevent patella instability. Arthrosc Tech 2:e125–e128
7. Kim SJ, Choi DH, Hwang BY (2012) The influence of posterolateral rotatory instability on ACL reconstruction: comparison between isolated ACL reconstruction and ACL reconstruction combined with posterolateral corner reconstruction. J Bone Joint Surg Am 94:253–259
8. Yoon KH, Lee JH, Bae DK, Song SJ, Chung KY, Park YW (2011) Comparison of clinical results of anatomic posterolateral corner reconstruction for posterolateral rotatory instability of the knee with or without popliteal tendon reconstruction. Am J Sports Med 39:2421–2428
9. Laprade RF, Wijdicks CA (2012) Surgical technique: development of an anatomic medial knee reconstruction. Clin Orthop Relat Res 470:806–814
10. Hui C, Roe J, Ferguson D, Waller A, Salmon L, Pinczewski L (2012) Outcome of anatomic transphyseal anterior cruciate ligament reconstruction in Tanner stage 1 and 2 patients with open physes. Am J Sports Med 40:1093–1098
11. Kennedy A, Coughlin DG, Metzger MF, Tang R, Pearle AD, Lotz JC, Feeley BT (2011) Biomechanical evaluation of pediatric anterior cruciate ligament reconstruction techniques. Am J Sports Med 39:964–971
12. Marx RG, Hetsroni I (2012) Surgical technique: medial collateral ligament reconstruction using Achilles allograft for combined knee ligament injury. Clin Orthop Relat Res 470:798–805
13. Spindler KP, Huston LJ, Wright RW, Kaeding CC, Marx RG, Amendola A, Parker RD, Andrish JT, Reinke EK, Harrell FE Jr, MOON Group, Dunn WR (2011) The prognosis and predictors of sports function and activity at minimum 6 years after anterior cruciate ligament reconstruction: a population cohort study. Am J Sports Med 39:348–359
14. Mirzatolooei F, Alamdari MT, Khalkhali HR (2013) The impact of platelet-rich plasma on the prevention of tunnel widening in anterior cruciate ligament reconstruction using quadrupled autologous hamstring tendon: a randomised clinical trial. Bone Joint J 95:65–69
15. Cervellin M, de Girolamo L, Bait C, Denti M, Volpi P (2012) Autologous platelet-rich plasma gel to reduce donor-site morbidity after patellar tendon graft harvesting for anterior cruciate ligament reconstruction: a randomized, controlled clinical study. Knee Surg Sports Traumatol Arthrosc 20:114–120

Anatomy and Biomechanics

2

Sven Scheffler

The peripheral compartments of the human knee joint can be divided into an anterior, posterior, medial, and lateral compartment.

The anterior compartment consists of the patellar tendon and Hoffa fat pad. Its main function is the force transduction of the upper leg via the extensor apparatus of the knee joint, i.e., the quadriceps tendon, to the lower leg via the patellar tendon. The posterior compartment mainly consists of the posterior capsule. The popliteus muscle runs posteriorly below the posterior capsule and inserts to the tibia above the soleus muscle. The tendons of the medial and lateral heads of the gastrocnemius muscle cross from distal to proximal the posterior periphery of the knee joint to attach to the distal femur and the lateral femoral condyle.

More important for overall knee function and often the location of soft tissue injuries are the medial and lateral periphery, which will be described in two separate sections.

2.1 Medial Periphery

2.1.1 Anatomy

The medial periphery of the human knee joint has been described to consist of three soft tissue layers [37]. The most superficial layer I is found subcutaneously and is formed by parts of the deep crural fascia. From proximal to distal it covers the sartorius and quadriceps muscle, blends anteriorly with the retinaculum, forming the deep crural fascia posteriorly, and runs distally toward the pes anserinus and tibial periosteum [41] (Fig. 2.1a).

Layer II is formed by the largest structure at the medial aspect of the knee, the superficial medial collateral ligament (sMCL) (Fig. 2.1b). It has been described to

S. Scheffler
COPV, Chirurgisch Orthopadischer Praxis Verbund, Berlin, Germany
e-mail: sven.scheffler@gmx.com

R. Rossi, F. Margheritini (eds.), *Knee Ligament Injuries*,
DOI 10.1007/978-88-470-5513-1_2, © Springer Verlag Italia 2014

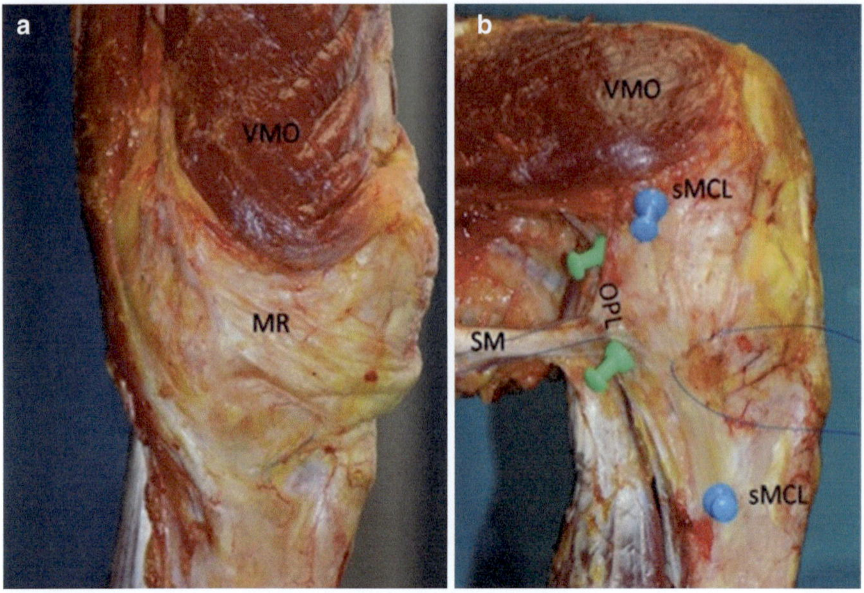

Fig. 2.1 (**a**, **b**) Superficial medial collateral ligament and posterior oblique ligament, *sMCL*: superficial medial collateral ligament; *MR*: medial retinaculum; *OPL*: oblique posterior ligament; *SM*: semimembranosus tendon; *VMO*: vastus medialis obliquus muscle

be between 10 and 12 cm long [23, 37]. It originates at the posterior-superior edge of the medial femoral epicondyle [20] and fans out to the tibial crest at 5–7 cm below the joint line, where two separate attachments can be found. The proximal tibial attachment is primarily to the anterior arm of the semimembranosus tendon. The larger distal bony attachment can be found anteriorly to the posteromedial crest of the tibia. Posterior to its tibial attachment, the sMCL blends within tibial expansions of the semimembranosus tendon. Anterior to the femoral attachment of the sMCL, it is continuous with the medial patellofemoral ligament (MPFL). The MPFL lies anterior to the medial capsule extra-articularly. It has been reported to have a length of approximately 55 mm and a varying width of 3–30 mm [1]. At the proximal edge of the MPFL, the vastus medialis obliquus muscle attaches. Often the MPFL can only be identified as a thickening of a fascial layer running from the proximal-medial edge of the patella to its femoral attachment between the posterior-superior site of the medial epicondyle and anterior-inferior site of the adductor tubercle [2, 20]. Soft tissue connections can be found to femoral attachments of the adductor magnus tendon and sMCL. Three muscles insert with their tendons to the posteromedial side of the knee joint. Most proximally, the adductor magnus tendon is attached in an osseous depression posterior-proximal to the adductor tubercle. At the distal-medial aspect of the adductor magnus tendon, a thick fascial expansion adheres to the medial gastrocnemius tendon, the capsular arm of the posterior oblique ligament, and the posteromedial capsule. More distally, the medial gastrocnemius tendon attaches in a depression proximal-posterior to the gastrocnemius tubercle. It has a thick fascial attachment to the adductor magnus tendon and a thin fascial attachment along its medial and posterior aspect to the capsular arm of the POL. Most distally, the semimembranosus tendon attachments are located on the medial and posteromedial parts of the tibia. The anterior arm of this distal insertion attaches deep to the proximal tibial attachment of the sMCL in an oval-shaped pattern distal to the tibial joint line. A direct arm connects to the posteromedial part of the tibia.

The medial joint capsule constitutes layer III. Posteriorly, its oblique fibers blend into layer II. It forms the deep MCL (dMCL) as a thickening below the sMCL, which spreads from the femoral condyle via the medial meniscus to the tibia. The dMCL shows a separate meniscotibial and meniscofemoral attachments, while blending with the sMCL posteriorly. The posteromedial capsule (PMC) is formed by dense tissue of layers II and III. Its femoral attachment site is at the adductor tubercle [12, 13, 24, 37]. Some authors identified a ligament-like structure within the PMC and termed it as the posterior oblique ligament (POL) [12, 13, 24]. The posterior border of the dMCL blends into the central arm of the POL, just posterior to the posterior edge of the sMCL. The POL is created by three fascial attachments to the semimembranosus tendon. It can be divided into a capsular, central, and superficial arm [12, 13]. The central and superficial arms blend into each other to form its femoral attachment posterior-inferior to the adductor tubercle and anterior-inferior to the gastrocnemius tubercle [20]. Distally, the thin superficial arm, which runs parallel to the posterior edge of the sMCL, merges with a distal expansion of the semimembranosus tendon. The strongest central part attaches distally to the posteromedial aspect of the medial meniscus, the posteromedial capsule, and the posteromedial aspect of the tibia [13, 20]. Anteriorly to the sMCL, layer III blends with layer I into the retinaculum.

The pes anserine tendons are situated between layers I and II–III and connect distally to the anteromedial aspect of the proximal part of the tibia. They consist of the sartorius, gracilis, and semitendinosus tendon in a proximal to distal fashion.

2.1.2 Biomechanics

The medial and posteromedial structures of the knee joint are loaded throughout the overall range of knee motion under valgus loads, internal and external rotation [6], as well as anterior and posterior drawer loads. There is a sharing response between the respective structures of the medial knee site, which act as primary and secondary restraint to various loads. The superficial medial collateral ligament (sMCL) has been identified as the primary restraint to valgus laxity of the knee [7, 17, 26] (Fig. 2.2). Griffith et al. [6] found that the sMCL does not function as one unit, but that its distal division was carrying larger loads than its proximal division, especially at flexion angles >20°, while the proximal sMCL was experiencing similar loads at all flexion angles. These differences in load transmission have been attributed to the different anatomy of the tibial attachments of the sMCL with the distal portion attaching directly to the tibia, therefore transmitting loads directly to the bone. In contrast, the

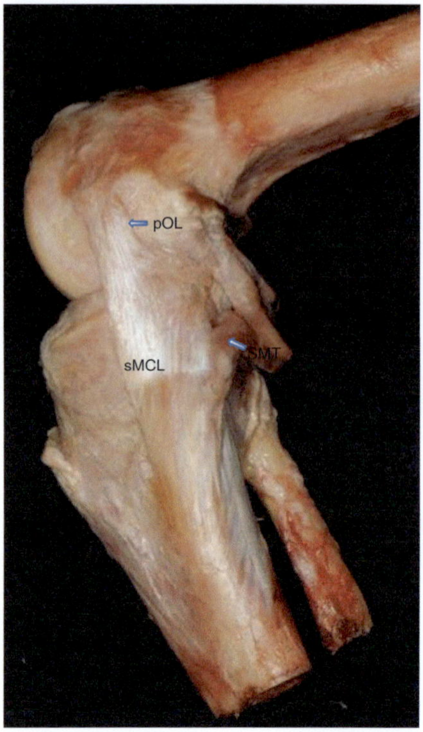

Fig. 2.2 Medial side knee anatomy. *POL* posterior oblique ligament, *sMCL* superior medial collateral ligament, *SMT* semimembranosus tendon

proximal part only has soft tissue adherences, which might disperse loads among the soft tissue structures more evenly. Mechanical testing of the distal and proximal sMCL has confirmed this different loading capacity with the distal MCL providing significantly higher structural properties (sMCL failure loads ≈ 500 N, stiffness ≈ 63 N/mm) than the proximal sMCL (failure load ≈ 85 N, stiffness ≈ 17 N/mm) [39]. It has been stated that this functional separation of the sMCL could have implications for future procedures for reconstruction of the sMCL [6]. The overall sMCL functions as a primary restraint to valgus loading with the knee joint in external rotation, especially when knee flexion increases [6, 32]. It acts as a secondary stabilizer to the ACL and PCL in restraining anterior and posterior translation of the tibia [6, 10, 28]. The posterior oblique ligament (POL) works as an important reinforcement of the posteromedial joint capsule (Fig. 2.2). It functions as a primary constraint to valgus loads toward extension [7, 13, 25, 27]. It has a failure load of around 250 N and provides a stiffness at around 40 N/mm [39]. While the sMCL primarily stabilizes at external rotation, the POL primarily provides stability at internal tibial rotation [6]. In internal rotation a reciprocal load response can be seen between the sMCL and POL with increasing flexion, suggesting a complementary relationship of these two structures [6]. Also, the POL works as a secondary restraint to anterior and posterior tibial translation throughout the range of knee motion [6] in the cruciate ligament intact and especially in the cruciate ligament-deficient knee joint [10, 17, 25, 27, 28]. The deep medial collateral ligament (dMCL) has significantly lower structural properties than the sMCL (failure load ≈ 100 N, stiffness ≈ 28 N/mm) [39]. It has been discovered as a secondary restraint to valgus loads with its meniscofemoral portion acting at all flexion angles and its meniscotibial portion working predominantly at 60° of flexion [5, 27, 40]. At flexion between 30° and 90°, the dMCL provides restraints against external rotation torque flexion [5, 40].

The semimembranosus tendon is known to produce direct stabilization of the posterior capsule through the oblique popliteal ligament and, indirectly, to add a synergistic action to the popliteus muscle through the fibrous expansion toward this muscle [14] (Fig. 2.2). As a dynamic stabilizer it provides additional stability to the posterior and posteromedial aspects of the knee, resisting internal torque and valgus stress with increasing knee flexion. Together with the popliteus muscle, it contributes to maintain posterior tibial stability. The attachments of the semimembranosus tendon to the posterior horn of the medial meniscus allow pulling of the meniscus backward in knee flexion, therefore protecting it from injury [13, 14].

The medial patellofemoral ligament (MPFL) is the primary restraint to lateral translation of the patella from extension until 30° of flexion, providing a mean tensile strength of 208 N [1]. While the medial retinaculum is tight at full extension, it slackens with flexion, contributing only around 11 % to overall lateral patella stabilization [4].The MPFL also guides the patella to engage centrally into the trochlea, underlining its importance for the alignment of the patellofemoral joint [3].

2.2 Lateral Periphery

2.2.1 Anatomy

Similar to the medial side, different tissue layers can be identified on the lateral side of the knee joint, which form the posterolateral complex (PLC).

Subcutaneously, the superficial layer of the *iliotibial band* can be found. It has a fascia-like structure and covers its deep fibers, which insert to the lateral supracondylar tubercle of the femur and blend into the lateral intramuscular septum [29, 33] (Fig. 2.3). Often, these layers are termed as "Kaplan fibers." Fibers of the iliotibial band run medially to the lateral gastrocnemius and plantaris muscles, while blending on the lateral aspect of the knee with the short head of the biceps femoris. These expansions of the iliotibial band, also called capsule-osseous layer, function as an anterolateral ligament of the knee [15, 22, 33]. Distally, the iliotibial band inserts onto the lateral tibial tuberosity at Gerdy's tubercle [33] (Fig. 2.3).

Medially, below the iliotibial band, the *biceps femoris muscle* with its long and short head tendinous insertions can be identified. The long head of the biceps tendon displays two tendinous insertions to the bone. The direct arm inserts onto the lateral aspect of the fibular styloid, covering the fibular insertion of the lateral collateral ligament (LCL). The anterior arm runs lateral to the LCL and inserts onto the lateral tibial plateau. Aponeurotic expansions connect the long and short heads of the biceps femoris to the posterolateral region of the LCL [33, 34]. The short head of the biceps femoris consists of three tendinous arms. The capsular arm runs from the main tendon to the

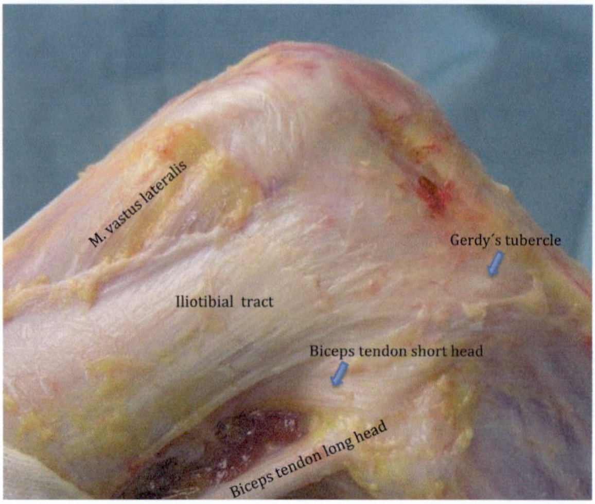

Fig. 2.3 Superficial structures of lateral compartment

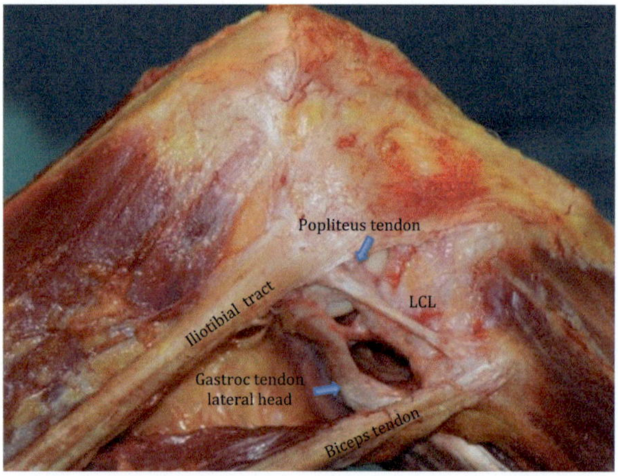

Fig. 2.4 Lateral collateral ligament

posterolateral joint capsule and inserts lateral to the tip of the fibular styloid. The fabellofibular ligament is formed by the distal edge of the capsular arm [33, 34]. The anterior arm inserts with the meniscotibial adhesions of the LCL at the proximolateral tibia. Often, ACL injuries are associated with an avulsion of this anterolateral aspect of the tibia, which has been termed a "Segond fracture" [31]. Identification of the biceps femoris tendon is imperative, since the peroneal nerve can be found posteriorly, 1.5–2 cm distal to the fibular styloid, advancing distally posterolateral to the fibular head.

The lateral collateral ligament (*LCL*) is an extra-articular structure of approximately 70 mm length. It inserts at the lateral aspect of the fibular head below the long head of the biceps tendon. Its femoral insertion can be found posterior to the lateral epicondyle (Fig. 2.4).

The popliteal sulcus can be found immediately distal to the femoral insertion of the LCL. It guides the *popliteus tendon* especially with increasing flexion, which inserts anterior and distal to the lateral epicondyle and the femoral insertion of the LCL as an intra-articular structure [15, 21, 38] (Fig. 2.4). The popliteus tendon courses distally with its intra-articular portion through the popliteal hiatus, providing branches to the lateral meniscus, the so-called popliteomeniscal fascicles. It acts as a dynamic stabilizer of the lateral meniscus. The popliteus tendon exits the knee joint through the coronary ligament, continuing to the popliteal fossa in the posterolateral corner. Multiple ligamentous insertions can be found here. The attachment of the popliteus tendon to the fibula comprises of the *anterior and posterior popliteofibular ligaments* [21]. The anterior ligament runs from the proximolateral musculotendinous junction medial to the LCL toward the fibula. The posterior ligament moves from the popliteus tendon to a distal region below the tip of the fibular styloid. Another attachment can be found from the anterior surface of the popliteus muscle to an area of the tibia, lateral to the fovea of the posterior cruciate ligament. This popliteotibial insertion is termed as a muscular aponeurotic attachment.

The combination of these attachments to the tibia, fibula, and lateral meniscus is called the *popliteus complex*. Finally, the popliteus tendon blends into its muscle in the popliteal fossa, with the popliteus muscle originating from the posteromedial aspect of the proximal tibia.

Proximal and posterior to the femoral insertion of the LCL, the thick tendon of the *lateral gastrocnemius muscle* can be easily identified. It blends into the meniscofemoral portion of the posterior capsule. The popliteofibular ligament shows expansions to the lateral head of the gastrocnemius muscle, therefore providing additional posterolateral stability.

The joint capsule has an anterior, lateral, and posterior portion on the lateral side of the knee joint. The anterior part spreads from the patellar tendon to the anterior border of the femoral insertion site of the popliteus tendon. From there, the lateral capsular part extends to the attachment of the lateral gastrocnemius tendon. The posterior capsule attaches to the femur proximal to the articular margin of the lateral femoral condyle.

Above the posterior capsule, the *oblique popliteal ligament* (ligament of Winslow) can be identified. It is formed by the coalescence of the oblique popliteal expansion of the semimembranosus and the capsular arm of the posterior oblique ligament. These two structures originate from the medial side of the knee, merge anterior to the medial head of the gastrocnemius, and form the oblique popliteal ligament. This ligament crosses the midsagittal plane of the knee at the level of the tibial insertion of the PCL and attaches to the inferomedial edge of the fabella and the lateral capsule [16, 30, 34].

2.2.2 Biomechanics

Multiple biomechanical studies exist that have analyzed the function and biomechanics of the lateral and posterolateral knee structures (PLC) [8, 9, 36, 38]. It is well accepted that these structures act as a primary restraint to varus loads and external tibial rotation and secondary to the PCL to posterior tibial translation.

The PLC has a strong interaction with the PCL. The PLC is an important stabilizer against posterior tibial translation near extension when the PCL is intact. In PCL-deficient knees, the posterolateral structures carry significantly higher loads under posterior tibial loading at extension and flexion, resulting in significantly higher posterior instability with additional PLC insufficiency [9]. Also, in situ forces of the PCL are greatly increased during posterior tibial loading with PLC structures deficient [9, 36]. The popliteus muscle is an important dynamic stabilizer against posterior knee instability, especially toward extension [8] when the PCL is intact. In a PCL-deficient knee joint, posterior tibial translation can be reduced by 36 % with loading of the popliteus tendon [8]. These findings underline the importance of identifying the exact extent of knee injury, especially on the lateral side, whether isolated or combined injuries are prevalent in order to decide what structures will have to be surgically addressed for restoration of normal posterior knee stability.

The lateral collateral ligament displays corresponding biomechanical function on the lateral side compared to the MCL on the medial side. It resists lateral joint opening (varus stress) at all flexion angles, experiencing the highest loading at 30° of flexion. It is assumed that around 300 N is required to rupture the LCL at this flexion angle [18]. The posterolateral structures provide additional stability against varus stress, especially with PCL injury [35, 36]. PLC insufficiency resulted into significantly increased varus rotation after PCL reconstruction [35, 36], pointing out the importance of meticulous diagnostics of any insufficiency of the various structures of the lateral periphery. The effect of the dynamic stabilizers of lateral knee periphery, the iliotibial band, biceps femoris muscle, and lateral gastrocnemius to resist varus loading plays only a minor role compared to the aforementioned structures [21].

It has been shown that the posterolateral complex and LCL are the primary restraints against external tibial rotation [8, 9, 11, 35]. The LCL is the dominating restraint from 0° to 30° of flexion. The popliteus tendon and popliteofibular ligament carry higher loads with increasing knee flexion up to 90° under external torque [19]. The intricate relationship of these structures with the PCL is underlined by the fact that cutting of the posterolateral structures in a PCL-deficient knee resulted into a markedly increased external rotational instability, most pronounced at 90° of flexion [11]. Major restraints to internal rotation of the knee joint are found on the medial side with structures of the PLC only providing little to no extra stability.

In summary, the understanding of the anatomy and biomechanics of the lateral structures of the knee joint are of utter importance to exactly understand what structures might be deficient. If surgical treatment is indicated, thorough knowledge of the anatomy will be a prerequisite to successfully restore normal function of the lateral and posterolateral structures of the knee joint.

References

1. Amis AA, Firer P, Mountney J, Senavongse W, Thomas NP (2003) Anatomy and biomechanics of the medial patellofemoral ligament. Knee 10:215–220
2. Baldwin JL (2009) The anatomy of the medial patellofemoral ligament. Am J Sports Med 37:2355–2361

3. Bicos J, Fulkerson JP, Amis A (2007) Current concepts review: the medial patellofemoral ligament. Am J Sports Med 35:484–492
4. Desio SM, Burks RT, Bachus KN (1998) Soft tissue restraints to lateral patellar translation in the human knee. Am J Sports Med 26:59–65
5. Griffith CJ, LaPrade RF, Johansen S, Armitage B, Wijdicks C, Engebretsen L (2009) Medial knee injury: part 1, static function of the individual components of the main medial knee structures. Am J Sports Med 37:1762–1770
6. Griffith CJ, Wijdicks CA, LaPrade RF, Armitage BM, Johansen S, Engebretsen L (2009) Force measurements on the posterior oblique ligament and superficial medial collateral ligament proximal and distal divisions to applied loads. Am J Sports Med 37:140–148
7. Grood ES, Noyes FR, Butler DL, Suntay WJ (1981) Ligamentous and capsular restraints preventing straight medial and lateral laxity in intact human cadaver knees. J Bone Joint Surg Am 63:1257–1269
8. Harner CD, Höher J, Vogrin TM, Carlin GJ, Woo SL (1998) The effects of a popliteus muscle load on in situ forces in the posterior cruciate ligament and on knee kinematics. A human cadaveric study. Am J Sports Med 26:669–673
9. Harner CD, Vogrin TM, Höher J, Ma CB, Woo SL (2000) Biomechanical analysis of a posterior cruciate ligament reconstruction. Deficiency of the posterolateral structures as a cause of graft failure. Am J Sports Med 28:32–39
10. Hinterwimmer S, Baumgart R, Plitz W (2002) Tension changes in the collateral ligaments of a cruciate ligament-deficient knee joint: an experimental biomechanical study. Arch Orthop Trauma Surg 122:454–458
11. Höher J, Harner CD, Vogrin TM, Baek GH, Carlin GJ, Woo SL (1998) In situ forces in the posterolateral structures of the knee under posterior tibial loading in the intact and posterior cruciate ligament-deficient knee. J Orthop Res 16:675–681
12. Hughston JC (1994) The importance of the posterior oblique ligament in repairs of acute tears of the medial ligaments in knees with and without an associated rupture of the anterior cruciate ligament. Results of long-term follow-up. J Bone Joint Surg Am 76:1328–1344
13. Hughston JC, Eilers AF (1973) The role of the posterior oblique ligament in repairs of acute medial (collateral) ligament tears of the knee. J Bone Joint Surg Am 55:923–940
14. Kaplan EB (1962) Some aspects of functional anatomy of the human knee joint. Clin Orthop 23:18–29
15. Kaplan EB (1958) The iliotibial tract; clinical and morphological significance. J Bone Joint Surg Am 40-A:817–832
16. Kaplan EB (1961) The fabellofibular and short lateral ligaments of the knee joint. J Bone Joint Surg Am 43-A:169–179
17. Kennedy JC, Fowler PJ (1971) Medial and anterior instability of the knee. An anatomical and clinical study using stress machines. J Bone Joint Surg Am 53:1257–1270
18. LaPrade RF (2005) Mechanical properties of the posterolateral structures of the knee. Am J Sports Med 33:1386–1391
19. LaPrade RF (2004) Force measurements on the fibular collateral ligament, popliteofibular ligament, and popliteus tendon to applied loads. Am J Sports Med 32:1695–1701
20. LaPrade RF, Engebretsen AH, Ly TV, Johansen S, Wentorf FA, Engebretsen L (2007) The anatomy of the medial part of the knee. J Bone Joint Surg Am 89:2000–2010
21. LaPrade RF, Ly TV, Wentorf FA, Engebretsen L (2003) The posterolateral attachments of the knee: a qualitative and quantitative morphologic analysis of the fibular collateral ligament, popliteus tendon, popliteofibular ligament, and lateral gastrocnemius tendon. Am J Sports Med 31:854–860
22. Lobenhoffer P, Posel P, Witt S, Piehler J, Wirth CJ (1987) Distal femoral fixation of the iliotibial tract. Arch Orthop Trauma Surg 106:285–290
23. Loredo R, Hodler J, Pedowitz R, Yeh LR, Trudell D, Resnick D (1999) Posteromedial corner of the knee: MR imaging with gross anatomic correlation. Skeletal Radiol 28:305–311
24. Müller W (1982) The knee. Form, function, and ligament reconstruction. Springer, New York BHN (eds)

25. Nielsen S, Rasmussen O, Ovesen J, Andersen K (1984) Rotatory instability of cadaver knees after transection of collateral ligaments and capsule. Arch Orthop Trauma Surg 103:165–169
26. Phisitkul P, James SL, Wolf BR, Amendola A (2006) MCL injuries of the knee: current concepts review. Iowa Orthop J 26:77–90
27. Robinson JR, Bull AMJ, Thomas RRD, Amis AA (2006) The role of the medial collateral ligament and posteromedial capsule in controlling knee laxity. Am J Sports Med 34:1815–1823
28. Sakane M, Livesay GA, Fox RJ, Rudy TW, Runco TJ, Woo SL (1999) Relative contribution of the ACL, MCL, and bony contact to the anterior stability of the knee. Knee Surg Sports Traumatol Arthrosc 7:93–97
29. Sanchez AR, Sugalski MT, LaPrade RF (2006) Anatomy and biomechanics of the lateral side of the knee. Sports Med Arthrosc 14:2–11
30. Seebacher JR, Inglis AE, Marshall JL, Warren RF (1982) The structure of the posterolateral aspect of the knee. J Bone Joint Surg Am 64:536–541
31. Segond P (1879) Recherches cliniques et expérimentales sur les épanchements sanguins du genou par entorse. Progres Med 7:297–299, 319–321, 340–341
32. Sims WF (2004) The posteromedial corner of the knee: medial-sided injury patterns revisited. Am J Sports Med 32:337–345
33. Terry GC, Hughston JC, Norwood LA (1986) The anatomy of the iliopatellar band and iliotibial tract. Am J Sports Med 14:39–45
34. Terry GC, LaPrade RF (1996) The biceps femoris muscle complex at the knee. Its anatomy and injury patterns associated with acute anterolateral-anteromedial rotatory instability. Am J Sports Med 24:2–8
35. Veltri DM, Deng XH, Torzilli PA, Warren RF, Maynard MJ (1995) The role of the cruciate and posterolateral ligaments in stability of the knee. A biomechanical study. Am J Sports Med 23:436–443
36. Vogrin TM, Höher J, Arøen A, Woo SL, Harner CD (2000) Effects of sectioning the posterolateral structures on knee kinematics and in situ forces in the posterior cruciate ligament. Knee Surg Sports Traumatol Arthrosc 8:93–98
37. Warren LF, Marshall JL (1979) The supporting structures and layers on the medial side of the knee: an anatomical analysis. J Bone Joint Surg Am 61:56–62
38. Watanabe Y, Moriya H, Takahashi K, Yamagata M, Sonoda M, Shimada Y, Tamaki T (1993) Functional anatomy of the posterolateral structures of the knee. Arthroscopy 9:57–62
39. Wijdicks CA, Ewart DT, Nuckley DJ, Johansen S, Engebretsen L, LaPrade RF (2010) Structural properties of the primary medial knee ligaments. Am J Sports Med 38:1638–1646
40. Wijdicks CA, Griffith CJ, LaPrade RF, Spiridonov SI, Johansen S, Armitage BM, Engebretsen L (2009) Medial knee injury: part 2, load sharing between the posterior oblique ligament and superficial medial collateral ligament. Am J Sports Med 37:1771–1776
41. Wymenga AB, Kats JJ, Kooloos J, Hillen B (2005) Surgical anatomy of the medial collateral ligament and the posteromedial capsule of the knee. Knee Surg Sports Traumatol Arthrosc 14:229–234

Acute Medial and Posteromedial Injury

3

Davide Edoardo Bonasia, Roberto Rossi, Federica Rosso, Umberto Cottino, Corrado Bertolo, and Filippo Castoldi

3.1 Introduction

Injuries to the medial collateral ligament (MCL) complex of the knee are the most common ligamentous lesions. A correct diagnosis, based on accurate physical examination and classification as well as imaging, is essential in treating these injuries. If correctly treated in the acute setting, these lesions usually do not result in medial chronic knee instability, with no need for more complex reconstruction procedures. A sound knowledge of the anatomy and biomechanics of the MCL complex is essential in achieving good results. The static portion of the MCL complex can be thought of as three linked components: the superficial MCL (sMCL), the deep MCL (dMCL), and the posterior oblique ligament (POL), which blends continuously with the first two. For precise description of the medial anatomy of the knee, the authors refer to the specific chapter of the present textbook. This chapter will review different aspects regarding MCL complex lesions, including injury pattern, clinical examination, classification, imaging, indications, conservative treatment, surgical anatomy, repair techniques, and results.

D.E. Bonasia, MD (✉) • C. Bertolo • F. Castoldi
Department of Orthopaedics and Traumatology, Azienda Ospedaliera Citta' della Salute e della Scienza, Presidio CTO- Maria Adelaide, Via Zuretti 29, Torino 10100, Italy
e-mail: davidebonasia@virgilio.it; corrado.bertolo@gmail.com; filippo.castoldi@unito.it

F. Rosso • U. Cottino
Department of Orthopaedics and Traumatology,
Azienda Ospedaliera Ordine Mauriziano, Largo Turati 62, Torino 10128, Italy
e-mail: federica.rosso@yahoo.it; umberto.cottino@gmail.com

R. Rossi
Department of Orthopaedics and Traumatology,
Mauriziano "Umberto I" Hospital, Largo Turati 62, Torino 10128, Italy
e-mail: rossir@fastwebnet.it

R. Rossi, F. Margheritini (eds.), *Knee Ligament Injuries*,
DOI 10.1007/978-88-470-5513-1_3, © Springer Verlag Italia 2014

3.2 Injury Pattern

Isolated injuries to the MCL complex primarily occur by two main mechanisms. The most common injury is a direct blow to the outside of the knee with the foot planted, producing direct valgus stress (i.e., in contact sports such as football, soccer, or rugby). Although the order in which the MCL complex structures become damaged is still debated, the sMCL and dMCL are thought to tear before the POL [1].

The second injury pattern involves a valgus stress coupled with tibial external rotation (i.e., in cutting and pivoting sports, such as basketball, soccer, and skiing). With this injury mechanism, it has been postulated that the POL and posteromedial corner are injured first, followed by the deep and superficial MCL. Both injury mechanisms place other knee structures at risk (mostly ACL, PCL, and menisci) [1].

Sims and Jacobson reviewed the charts of 93 knees with operatively treated isolated and combined medial-sided knee injuries and described the associated medial injury patterns. The authors found that the POL was torn in 99 % of the cases, the sMCL in 33 %, the dMCL in 25 %, the semimembranosus tendinous expansions in 70 %, the meniscotibial and meniscofemoral ligaments in 83 %, and the meniscus in 43 %. Associated ACL injuries were found in 73 knees and associated PCL injuries in 2 knees. The POL had a focal lesion in 71 % of the cases (femoral 32 %, interstitial 12 %, and tibial 27 %) and a multifocal lesion in 29 % of the cases. Out of 93 knees, the sMCL had a focal lesion in 27 % of the cases (femoral 11 %, interstitial 1 %, and tibial 15 %) and a multifocal lesion in 6 % of the cases. Meniscal injuries had been recorded in 40 knees (20 peripheral tears, 17 body tears, and 3 tears that involved both the body and periphery) [2].

3.3 Classification, Clinical Examination, and Imaging

In the diagnosis of MCL lesions, the authors prefer the Fetto and Marshall classification. This classification divides medial-sided knee injuries into grade 1 (no valgus laxity), grade 2 (valgus laxity at 30° of flexion), and grade 3 (valgus laxity at 0° and 30°) [3]. The stability of the knee is then tested in all planes in order to evaluate anteroposterior, lateral, and rotational instability.

By definition, patients with medial-sided injuries have increased laxity with valgus stress. The examiner applies a valgus stress to the knee at both 0° and 30° of flexion. For isolated sMCL injuries, the greatest joint space opening occurs with the knee in 30° of flexion [4]. Joint space opening with the knee fully extended indicates an injury to the capsule, the POL, or both. Grade III MCL injuries are frequently associated with injury to another ligament (mostly the ACL) [5].

Other physical examination maneuvers combine rotation with various amounts of knee flexion in an attempt to discriminate between MCL and MCL/PMC injuries. One of the most common involves a valgus stress to the knee in 30° of flexion with the foot externally rotated [5]. The presence of anteromedial rotary instability (AMRI) is indicative of PMC injury. AMRI is detected by performing the anterior drawer test with the tibia both in neutral and in external rotation. Increased translation with the tibia in external rotation is indicative of AMRI [6, 7].

Increased external rotation and AMRI indicate injury to the PMC and possibly to the ACL as well.

Weight-bearing radiographs of the knee are obtained in anteroposterior and lateral views. If valgus malalignment is present, a weight-bearing long leg radiograph is obtained. MRI is helpful in diagnosing associated bone and soft tissue injuries (anterior and posterior cruciate ligaments, posterolateral corner, and menisci) as well as determining the location and extent of medial/posteromedial ligamentous injuries. However, it has been shown that MRI tends to overestimate injury to ligamentous structures [8].

3.4 Indications

In the acute setting (<3 weeks), the treatment of isolated and combined grade I–II injuries is mostly conservative [9, 10], but significant controversies exist regarding the treatment of isolated and combined grade III lesions [11, 12]. In case of isolated grade III injuries, conservative treatment can be considered with varus or neutral alignment. On the other hand, surgery is indicated in case of severe valgus alignment, bony avulsions, and intra-articular MCL entrapment [13].

In case of combined ACL and grade III MCL injuries, the treatment is controversial. The first option is to conservatively treat the MCL and delay the ACL reconstruction. If medial opening >4 mm compared to contralateral knee is present after ACL reconstruction, MCL reconstruction or capsular procedures should be considered. Otherwise, an early ACL reconstruction can be performed, with subsequent conservative MCL treatment. Lastly, acute MCL repair with concomitant ACL reconstruction can be performed.

The treatment is controversial also in case of combined ACL, PCL, and grade III MCL injuries. The different options include (1) conservative MCL + delayed PCL/ACL reconstruction, (2) acute MCL repair/PCL reconstruction + delayed ACL reconstruction, and (3) acute MCL repair/ACL/PCL reconstruction [13].

3.5 Conservative Treatment

When adopting conservative treatment for MCL complex lesions, the authors' preferred protocol is as described by Edson [14].

Grade I MCL injuries. Weight bearing as tolerated with crutches if necessary. Active ROM exercises as soon as tolerated. Active strengthening exercises as tolerated. Progress to agility, proprioceptive, and sport-specific drills as tolerated. Return to sports when strength, agility, and proprioception are equal to the uninvolved side [14].

Grade II MCL injuries. Long leg brace for ambulation with weight bearing as tolerated with crutches. Brace may be locked in extension for 1–2 weeks depending upon pain, valgus opening, and anatomic alignment. Crutches can be discontinued when patient attains a nonantalgic gait. Active ROM exercises are started immediately. Electrical stimulation to the quadriceps, quad sets, and single leg raise are initiated immediately. Long leg brace is opened at the end of the third week and full weight bearing is encouraged. Severe grade II injuries may require 6 weeks of bracing. Once full ROM and functional strength is attained, proprioceptive and agility drills can be initiated [14].

Grade III MCL injuries. Immobilization in long leg brace locked in extension for 3–6 weeks depending on anatomic alignment. Nonweight bearing for 3 weeks in patients with valgus alignment. Toe-touch weight bearing for neutral or varus. Immediate ROM out of the brace two to three times a day for neutral or varus alignment, after 3 weeks for patients with valgus. Strengthening is done throughout the 6-week period in the form of quad sets, single leg raise, and electrical stimulation. Closed chain exercises are initiated at the appropriate time depending upon patient's weight-bearing status [14].

3.6 Surgical Anatomy

The anatomy of the medial side of the knee has been extensively described by LaPrade and colleagues (Figs. 3.1 and 3.2) [15]. The structures of the medial side of the knee include (1) bony landmarks (medial epicondyle, adductor tubercle,

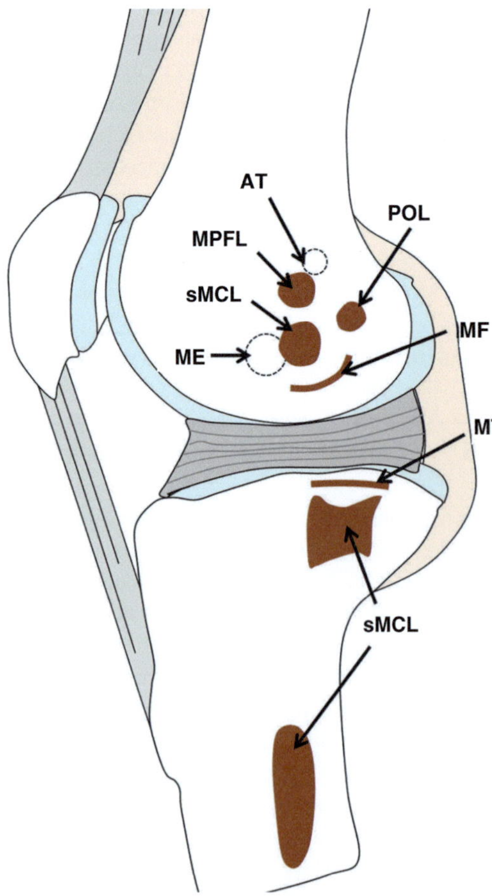

Fig. 3.1 Medial view of the knee: attachment sites (Redrawn from Bonasia et al. [13]). *AT* adductor tubercle, *ME* medial epicondyle, *sMCL* superficial medial collateral ligament, *MPFL* medial patellofemoral ligament, *POL* posterior oblique ligament, *MF* meniscofemoral ligament, *MT* meniscotibial ligament

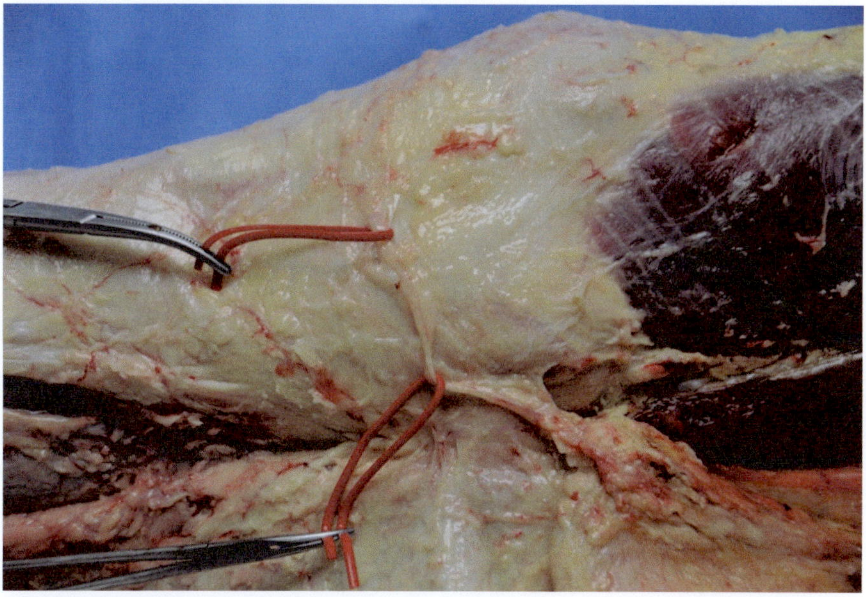

Fig. 3.2 Saphenous nerve and infrapatellar branch of the saphenous nerve

gastrocnemius tubercle on the femur, medial tibial plateau, medial aspect of the patella), (2) ligaments (superficial medial collateral ligament, deep medial collateral ligament, posterior oblique ligament, medial patellofemoral ligament, posteromedial capsule), and (3) tendons (adductor magnus, medial head of the gastrocnemius, semimembranosus, and pes anserinus).

The sMCL (Figs. 3.1 and 3.3) has 1 femoral and 2 tibial attachments (proximal and distal). The femoral attachment has an oval shape and is located 3.2 mm proximal and 4.8 mm posterior to the medial epicondyle. The proximal tibial attachment is primarily to soft tissues, mainly to the anterior arm of the semimembranosus tendon. The distal tibial attachment of the sMCL is just anterior to the posteromedial crest of the tibia. The average distance of the proximal tibial attachment is 12.2 mm from the tibial joint line. The average distance of the distal tibial attachment is 94.8 mm from the femoral attachment and 61.2 mm from the tibial joint line. The average distance from the distal tibial attachment to proximal tibial attachment is 49.2 mm [15].

The dMCL (Figs. 3.1 and 3.3) is a thickening of the medial joint capsule. The dMCL consists of the meniscofemoral (MF) and meniscotibial (MT) ligaments. The MF ligament is longer than the MT ligament and its attachment is located 15.1 mm posterior and distal to the medial epicondyle. The MT ligament is shorter and thicker and attaches just distal (3.2 mm average) to the cartilage of the medial tibial plateau [15].

The posterior oblique ligament (POL) consists of three fascial attachments (Figs. 3.1 and 3.3): superficial, central (tibial), and capsular. The three attachments

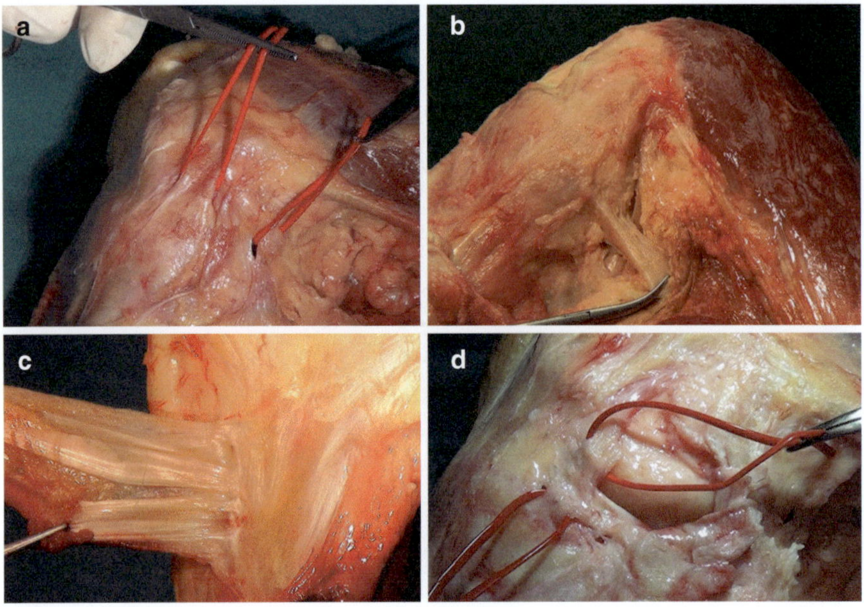

Fig. 3.3 Anatomy of the medial side of the knee. (**a**) sMCL (*left loop*) and POL (*right loop*). (**b**) Semimembranosus tendon (held by the Kelly clamp). (**c**) Distal sMCL insertion (after detachment of the pes anserinus). (**d**) dMCL with meniscofemoral (proximal loop) and meniscotibial (distal loop) ligaments

course off the distal aspect of the semimembranosus tendon mainly, but also off the medial meniscus, posteromedial tibia, and medial head of the gastrocnemius. On the average, the POL attaches on the femur 7.7 mm distal and 6.4 mm posterior to the adductor tubercle and 1.4 mm distal and 2.9 mm anterior to the gastrocnemius tubercle [15].

3.7 Repair Technique

Examination under anesthesia is performed to completely assess the injury. Arthroscopy can be used to rule out any other associated lesions and determine the site of the dMCL injury. In the acute setting, arthroscopy should be performed quickly and with gravity inflow, to minimize fluid extravasation. A hockey stick (or longitudinal) incision is made from the medial proximal tibia to the medial femoral epicondyle, curving posteriorly in line with the intermuscular septum. For isolated distal or proximal detachment repair, a more limited approach can be used. In the case of combined treatment of acute complete MCL tear and an ACL tear, exposure of the MCL is easier if approached through a separate medial incision as opposed to extending the tibial incision for the ACL reconstruction. Attention should be paid to preserve the saphenous nerve (Fig. 3.2). The crural and sartorial

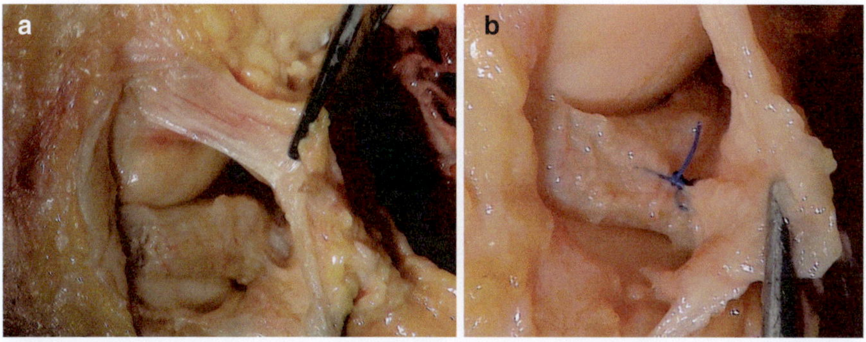

Fig. 3.4 (**a**) Capsular detachment of the medial meniscus. (**b**) Repair of the capsular detachment with an open technique

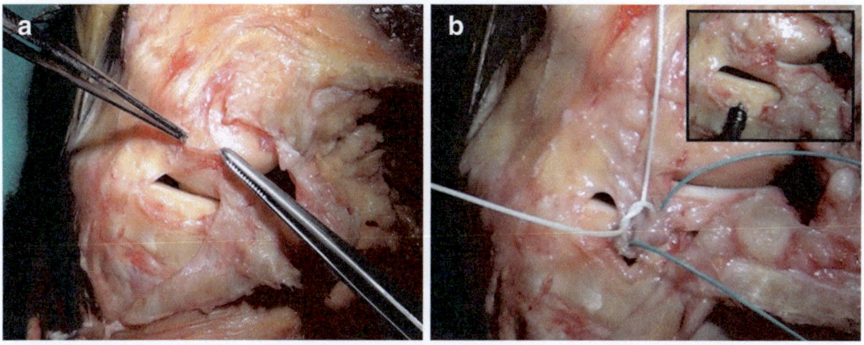

Fig. 3.5 Repair technique. (**a**, **b**) A meniscotibial ligament tear repaired with suture anchor fixation

fascia is incised longitudinally. Hematoma is removed. The injured structures are then identified [16].

The injured structures are identified and should be repaired from the deepest structure outward. A peripheral tear of the medial meniscus is commonly seen and repaired with an open technique (Fig. 3.4) [16]. A meniscofemoral ligament tear can be directly repaired using sutures alone or suture anchors (Fig. 3.5). Suture anchor fixation is preferred for meniscotibial ligament tear. If injured, the POL is repaired by direct suture back to the femur. Repair of the deep structures is completed with the knee held in varus and full extension [16].

Femoral avulsion of the sMCL (Fig. 3.6) leaves the best tissue for repair using suture anchors, staples, or a screw/washer. However, repair in this location is associated with postoperative stiffness, more than in other locations [17]. This is due to the great importance of the femoral isometric point of the sMCL. It is difficult to attach the sMCL back to the femoral isometric point, due to soft tissue retraction. Acute complete avulsions off of the tibia can be repaired, using either suture anchors or staples [16].

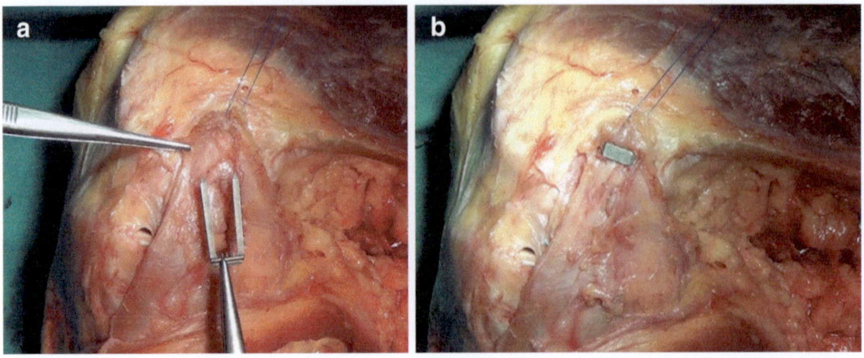

Fig. 3.6 Repair technique. (**a**, **b**) Femoral avulsion of the sMCL repaired using Richard's staples

The semimembranosus portion of the POL can be repaired with interrupted absorbable sutures and sutured to the posterior border of the MCL in a pants-over-vest fashion. Occasionally, mid-substance and tibial-sided injuries require augmentation, due to the poor soft tissue quality. The sMCL is fixed at 30° of knee flexion [16]. Finally, the tourniquet is deflated and inspection and control of potential excessive bleeding from the inferior medial geniculate artery and its branches is performed. A compressive dressing is applied postoperatively.

Postoperatively, the patient is kept in a hinged knee brace with protected weight bearing. Passive range of motion from 0 to 90° is begun immediately. Hyperextension and flexion over 90° should be avoided during the first 2 weeks. Isometric and closed kinetic chain strengthening are allowed immediately. Full range of motion is allowed 2 weeks after surgery, and full weight bearing is allowed 6 weeks after surgery. Return to sports is generally allowed 6 months after surgery.

3.8 Results

Good results have been reported for the conservative treatment of grade I and II MCL complex tears [18, 19].

Several authors reported good results after conservative management of isolated grade III medial-sided knee injuries [3, 20–23]. As a consequence, many orthopedic surgeons initially treat isolated MCL complex injuries nonoperatively regardless of the grade.

Indelicato prospectively evaluated the results of conservative treatment (20 knees) and primary repair (16 knees) in 36 patients with isolated grade III MCL complex injuries [24]. The percentage of patients with good to excellent stability after treatment was higher in the operative group (94 % vs. 85 %). However, no functional significance was found between the two groups in combined objective-subjective scoring. Patients treated nonoperatively started range of motion sooner and completed the rehabilitation program significantly faster. Notably, no MCL complex was considered normal after treatment in either group, nor did it ever provide the same firmness as the uninjured side.

In 1983, Hughston and Barrett [25] reported the results of acute MCL complex repair in 89 patients with anteromedial instability (2+ or more). With an average follow-up of 7.8 years, 94 % of the patients returned to preinjury level of performance.

In 1994, Hughston [26] reported the results of acute MCL complex repair in 40 patients with anteromedial instability (2+ or more), at an average 20-year follow-up. Ninety-three percent of the patients had good results and only a 7 % rate of failure was reported.

Conclusions

Grade I and II MCL complex lesions can be successfully managed with conservative treatment.

Although controversies still exist regarding the correct treatment for grade III MCL complex lesions, the treatment should be based on different factors, including patient's age and activity level, lower limb alignment, and concomitant lesions to other structures. Therefore, the treatment should be tailored on each specific case.

References

1. Marchant MH Jr, Tibor LM, Sekiya JK, Hardaker WT Jr, Garrett WE Jr, Taylor DC (2011) Management of medial-sided knee injuries, part 1: medial collateral ligament. Am J Sports Med 39:1102–1113
2. Sims WF, Jacobson KE (2004) The posteromedial corner of the knee: medial-sided injury patterns revisited. Am J Sports Med 32:337–345
3. Fetto JF, Marshall JL (1978) Medial collateral ligament injuries of the knee: a rationale for treatment. Clin Orthop 132:206–218
4. Fanelli GC, Harris JD (2006) Surgical treatment of acute medial collateral ligament and posteromedial corner injuries of the knee. Sports Med Arthrosc 14:78–83
5. Tibor LM, Marchant MH Jr, Taylor DC, Hardaker WT Jr, Garrett WE Jr, Sekiya JK (2011) Management of medial-sided knee injuries, part 2: posteromedial corner. Am J Sports Med 39:1332–1340
6. Robinson JR, Bull AMJ, Thomas RR, Amis AA (2006) The role of the medial collateral ligament and posteromedial capsule in controlling knee laxity. Am J Sports Med 34:1815–1823
7. Bauer KL, Stannard JP (2013) Surgical approach to the posteromedial corner: indications, technique, outcomes. Curr Rev Musculoskelet Med 6:124–131
8. Lonner JH, Dupuy DE, Siliski JM (2000) Comparison of magnetic resonance imaging with operative findings in acute traumatic dislocations of the adult knee. J Orthop Trauma 14:183–186
9. Holden DL, Eggert AW, Butler JE (1983) The nonoperative treatment of grades I and II medial collateral ligament injuries to the knee. Am J Sports Med 11:340–344. 36
10. Indelicato PA, Hermansdorfer J, Huegel M (1990) Nonoperative management of complete tears of the medial collateral ligament of the knee in intercollegiate football players. Clin Orthop Relat Res 256:174–177

11. Klimkiewicz JJ, Petrie RS, Harner CD (2000) Surgical treatment of combined injury to anterior cruciate ligament, posterior cruciate ligament and medial structures. Clin Sports Med 19:479–492
12. Levy BA, Fanelli GC, Whelan DB, Stannard JP, MacDonald PA, Boyd JL, et al, Knee Dislocation Study Group (2009) Controversies in the treatment of knee dislocation and multiligament reconstruction. J Am Acad Orthop Surg 17:197–206
13. Bonasia DE, Bruzzone M, Dettoni F, Marmotti A, Blonna D, Castoldi F, Gasparetto F, D'Elicio D, Collo G, Rossi R (2012) Treatment of medial and posteromedial knee instability: indications, techniques, and review of the results. Iowa Orthop J 32:173–183
14. Edson CJ (2006) Conservative and postoperative rehabilitation of isolated and combined injuries of the medial collateral ligament. Sports Med Arthrosc 14:105–110
15. LaPrade RF, Engebretsen AH, Ly TV, Johansen S, Wentorf FA, Engebretsen L (2007) The anatomy of the medial part of the knee. J Bone Joint Surg Am 89:2000–2010
16. Phisitkul P, James SL, Wolf BR, Amendola A (2006) MCL injuries of the knee: current concepts review. Iowa Orthop J 26:77–90
17. Robins AJ, Newman AP, Burks RT (1993) Postoperative return of motion in anterior cruciate ligament and medial collateral ligament injuries. The effect of medial collateral ligament rupture location. Am J Sports Med 21(1):20–25
18. Derscheid GL, Garrick JG (1981) Medial collateral ligament injuries in football: nonoperative management of grade I and grade II sprains. Am J Sports Med 9:365–368
19. Lundberg M, Messner K (1996) Long-term prognosis of isolated partial medial collateral ligament ruptures: a ten-year clinical and radiographic evaluation of a prospectively observed group of patients. Am J Sports Med 24:160–163
20. Jones RE, Henley B, Francis P (1986) Nonoperative management of isolated grade III collateral ligament injury in high school football players. Clin Orthop Relat Res 213:137–140
21. Reider B, Sathy MR, Talkington J, Blyznak N, Kollias S (1993) Treatment of isolated medial collateral ligament injuries in athletes with early functional rehabilitation: a five-year follow-up study. Am J Sports Med 22:470–477
22. Sandberg R, Balkfors B, Nilsson B, Westlin N (1987) Operative versus nonoperative treatment of recent injuries to the ligaments of the knee. J Bone Joint Surg Am 69:1120–1126
23. Shelbourne KD, Porter DA (1992) Anterior cruciate ligament–medial collateral ligament injury: nonoperative management of the medial collateral ligament tears with anterior cruciate ligament reconstruction. A preliminary report. Am J Sports Med 20:283–286
24. Indelicato PA (1983) Non-operative treatment of complete tears of the medial collateral ligament of the knee. J Bone Joint Surg Am 65:323–329
25. Hughston JC, Barrett GR (1983) Acute anteromedial rotatory instability. Long-term results of surgical repair. J Bone Joint Surg Am 65:145–153
26. Hughston JC (1994) The importance of the posterior oblique ligament in repairs of acute tears of the medial ligaments in knees with and without an associated rupture of the anterior cruciate ligament. Results of long-term follow-up. J Bone Joint Surg Am 76:1328–1344

Acute Lateral and Posterolateral Injury

4

Mark D. Miller and Matthew T. Burrus

4.1 Approach

Injuries to the posterolateral corner (PLC) of the knee have become more commonly recognized in recent years. In patients with an acute hemarthrosis following a knee injury, LaPrade et al. found a 9.1 % incidence of damage to the PLC on MRI [1]. Another study revealed MRI evidence of PLC damage in 68 % of operative tibial plateau fractures [2]. It is important to appreciate that PLC injuries are often associated with loss to other static and dynamic restraints around the knee, as one study showed isolated PLC damage in only 2 % of soft tissue knee injuries [3]. While the vast majority of these PLC injuries do not require surgery or even bracing, this data should heighten the clinician's awareness of their prevalence. Thus, a thorough workup involving a detailed physical exam and advanced imaging is indicated to fully characterize the injury prior to choosing a management option.

The typical mechanism of injury to the PLC includes a hyperextension injury (contact or noncontact), varus force to the knee, or direct trauma to the anteromedial knee. A thorough neurovascular exam is mandatory, paying special attention to foot dorsiflexion and digit extension and to the sensory exam in the superficial and deep peroneal nerve distributions. The incidence of peroneal nerve dysfunction after a PLC injury was found to be 15 % by LaPrade et al. in 1997, and it is important to know and document the patient's nerve function prior to going to the operating room [4]. Additionally, perfusion to the foot should be included in the consult note, including descriptors such as color, temperature, dopperable versus palpable pulses, and the ankle-brachial index (ABI) if appropriate. If there is significant injury to other ligamentous structures around the knee, then a knee dislocation must be suspected, even if the initial radiographs show a well-reduced knee. There must be a

M.D. Miller, MD (✉) • M.T. Burrus
Department of Orthopaedic Surgery, University of Virginia,
400 Ray C. Hunt Drive, Suite 300, 800159, Charlottesville, VA 22908, USA
e-mail: mdm3p@hscmail.mcc.virginia.edu; mtb3u@hscmail.mcc.virginia.edu

R. Rossi, F. Margheritini (eds.), *Knee Ligament Injuries*,
DOI 10.1007/978-88-470-5513-1_4, © Springer Verlag Italia 2014

high suspicion for a vascular injury in these situations with additional noninvasive and/or invasive studies performed and possibly vascular surgery involvement.

There are several physical maneuvers that are important in characterizing the presence and severity of injury to posterolateral structures. Measuring the patient's knee range of motion (ROM) is extremely important as a reliable predictor of postoperative ROM. A short period of physical therapy can decrease swelling, improve ROM, and should be considered before surgery is undertaken. The first and most basic exam involves testing varus and valgus laxity at 0° and 30° of flexion. Injury to the lateral structures increase the joint space when a varus force is applied; if isolated, then only opening at 30° is seen. If the knee opens laterally in full extension as well, then one must suspect an injury to one or both of the cruciates. Next, testing the ACL with the Lachman's test and then the PCL at 90° of flexion with the posterior drawer test further illuminates the status of the soft tissue restraints. A 3+ posterior drawer (>10 mm of side-to-side difference) is indicative of a combined PCL/PLC injury [5].

Rotatory testing is also important in characterizing PLC injuries. The dial, or external rotation asymmetry test, measures the thigh-foot angle when the tibia is externally rotated. When compared to the uninjured side, greater than 15° of asymmetry is indicative of deficient posterolateral restraints. If significant asymmetry is seen at 30° of knee flexion and not 90°, then PLC structures are torn, but the PCL is spared. However, it should be noted that this does not rule out an ACL injury. If significant asymmetry is seen at both 30° and 90° of knee flexion, then there is likely a combined PCL/PLC injury. This test can be performed with the patient either prone or supine. The posterolateral drawer test also aims to uncover combined PCL/PLC disruptions by applying a posterior force with the foot externally rotated. In a positive test, the knee displaces posteriorly and rotates laterally. For the reverse pivot shift test, a valgus force is applied to the knee while it is taken from a flexed to extended position. If a clunk is felt or visualized, then you are noticing the tibia moving from a posteriorly subluxed position to a reduced position as the iliotibial (IT) band becomes a knee extensor. An exam should be performed when the patient is initially seen in clinic, but an exam under anesthesia prior to incision when the patient is not guarding is extremely helpful as well.

As in all other orthopedic disorders, imaging plays a crucial role in the management of PLC injuries. Plain radiographs are usually not particularly useful unless an arcuate sign is noted in which there is an avulsion injury to the proximal fibula by the biceps femoris, popliteofibular ligament (PFL), or lateral collateral ligament (LCL) (Fig. 4.1). However, we have found that stress radiographs, similar to a physical exam, provide information regarding clinically relevant laxity. To isolate the collateral ligaments, we place the knee over a foam triangle and provide varus and valgus stresses at 20–30° of flexion. When compared to the contralateral side, greater than 2.7–4 mm of difference is suggestive of a Grade III LCL and PLC injury [7]. When testing the posterior drawer, one can quantify the posterior translation of the tibia on a lateral X-ray, and greater than 10 mm side-to-side difference indicates a combined PCL/PLC injury [5]. This posterior force of 15D_AN can be applied with a TELOS Stress Device (Telos GmbH, Marburg, Germany) or with lead gloves.

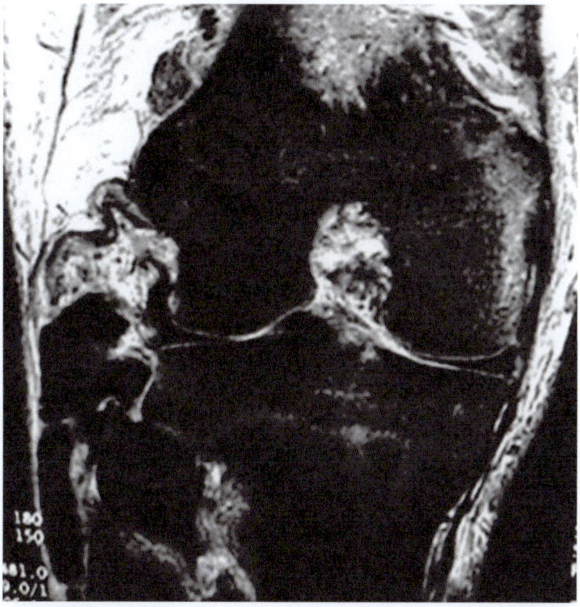

Fig. 4.1 Coronal MRI showing significant disruption to the posterolateral corner structures (This image was published in Miller et al. [6], with permission)

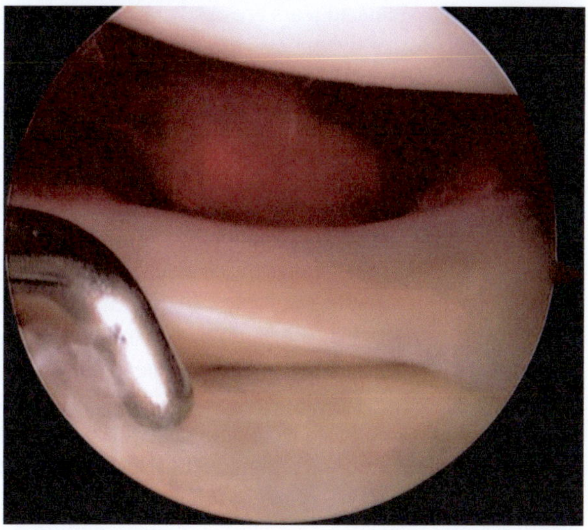

Fig. 4.2 Arthroscopic view of a lateral capsular avulsion off of the femur (i.e., the meniscus remains with the tibia) as well as a positive drive-through sign

MRI scans are obtained on almost all patients to provide more information and further clarify as to what to expect during surgery (Fig. 4.2). They are especially useful if a ligament or tendon is avulsed without a large enough bony fragment to be seen on X-ray as this can direct your dissection intraoperatively. All of the above physical exam tests are important, as an MRI can misrepresent injuries and do not elucidate the clinical relevance of a "high-grade tear" or of "ligament attenuation." MRI images should be used in conjunction with and not in lieu of a physical exam.

Once the patient and clinician have decided on surgical management, it is of our opinion that acutely managing these injuries results in superior outcomes, and this has been validated in multiple studies [8, 9]. We usually define as acute as surgically addressing the injury within 2 weeks.

4.2 Surgical Technique

In order to access the knee posterolateral structures, it is important to have the appropriate patient positioning and OR table setup. The patient is positioned supine on a radiolucent OR table with a bump under the ipsilateral buttock. Another option includes a lazy lateral position with a bean bag positioner. If the PCL is being reconstructed concomitantly with an inlay technique, then a lateral decubitus position is used. An AFO-type leg holder and nonsterile tourniquet are placed on the operative extremity.

Each case includes an arthroscopic evaluation of the joint to fully characterize the intra-articular pathology. A drive-through sign (>1 cm of joint space opening) is often present in the lateral compartment, and it should be noted if the meniscus remains close to the tibia or femur as this will give the surgeon an idea from which side the joint capsule may be avulsed and, therefore, which side needs to be repaired [10] (Fig. 4.3). Meniscal tears are easily seen as the wide joint space allows uncommon visualization of the entire lateral meniscus. These are usually repaired using an inside-out or open technique utilizing the open lateral incision which is soon to be developed. Prior to the initial diagnostic arthroscopy, we always perform an initial dissection of the lateral knee in order to allow for egress of the arthroscopic fluid. This help to greatly reduce the risk for iatrogenic leg compartment syndrome.

After drawing out the lateral and posterolateral landmarks (fibular head, Gerdy's tubercle, tibial tubercle, posterior edge of the iliotibial (IT) band), an 8–10 cm vertical incision is centered at the joint line just anterior to the fibula. The planned incision is drawn out in extension and is made with the knee in 90° of flexion. The subcutaneous tissue is dissected to expose the IT band and the biceps tendon. At this point, it is important to identify and protect the peroneal nerve which is located just posterior to the biceps. In order to have safe access to the proximal fibula during the reconstruction, you must carefully dissect out the nerve around the neck of the fibula. The nerve is protected throughout the remainder of the case. Next, the interval between the iliotibial tract (posterior 1/3 of the iliotibial band) and the biceps is developed to allow identification of the lateral collateral ligament, popliteofibular ligament, and popliteus tendon. A second interval (slightly anterior and distal) is found between the iliotibial band and iliotibial tract where the lateral femoral condyle can be accessed. The second interval allows visualization of the popliteus and LCL. Using this approach, the peroneal nerve is easily retracted posteriorly and out of the surgical field. Alternative approaches have been described such as making multiple deep windows or intervals to access particular structures. We have found that a larger single incision with two adequately sized intervals provides better access to the deep structures and allows the surgeon to continuously keep an eye on the peroneal nerve.

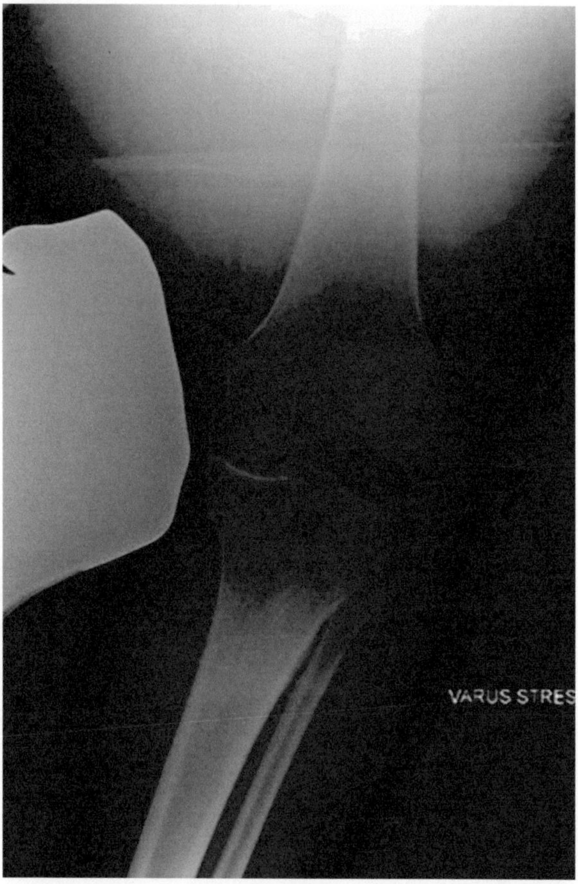

Fig. 4.3 AP radiograph with a varus stress applied with significant lateral joint space opening with displacement of the avulsed fibular head (i.e., arcuate sign)

When acutely addressing these injuries (ideally within 2 weeks), individual structures are able to be identified before the whole area becomes encased in scar tissue. These ligaments and tendons should be dissected out to see if they are amenable to repair, to help locate accurate insertions and origins for graft placement, and to provide local native ligament to augment reconstructions. Although repair is often possible in these acute situations, it is sometimes very difficult to achieve secure fixation as the damaged tissue has been stretched to failure, and thus the ends are often frayed and do not hold suture well. One exception to that rule is seen with body avulsion injuries as seen radiographically as the arcuate sign (Fig. 4.3). This type of failure is particularly amenable to anatomic repair with suture anchors or, depending on the bony fragment size, screw and washer constructs. If secured and immobilized appropriately postoperatively, avulsion injuries reliably heal because of the strong bone to bone reparative process. It is important to remove all soft tissue intervening between the bony fragments and to not entrap the peroneal nerve during fixation around the fibular head. Additionally, lateral meniscal tears are commonly seen in these injuries and should be repaired when possible although techniques for this procedure will not be discussed in this chapter. Primary repair of mid-substance injuries of the LCL with sutures, or reattachment of soft tissue avulsions with suture anchors, heal less dependably due to the watershed nature of this region, the quality of the damaged tissue, and less secure fixation methods. An acute repair of the LCL in an end-to-end fashion augmented with a strip of the long head of the biceps has been described, and Coobs et al. demonstrated that reconstruction of the LCL has been shown to be biomechanically superior to repair if no augmentation is added [11, 12]. It is for these reasons that reconstruction is the preferred technique even in acute injuries. In acute PLC injuries, Stannard et al. had a 37 % failure rate when repaired compared to 9 % when reconstructed using the modified 2-tail technique [13]. In our experience with these situations, more reliable immediate and long-term stability is achieved by using a soft tissue graft to reconstruct the torn structure than by repairing.

There are many techniques which have been described to reconstruct the posterolateral corner. They are often divided into anatomic and nonanatomic, with non-anatomic being mainly of historical interest. Commonly used techniques include the Muller popliteal bypass procedure, Larson figure of eight PLC reconstruction, two-tail PLC reconstruction, three-tail PLC reconstruction, and LaPrade PLC reconstruction. There are small variations between these procedures, but all rely on free soft tissue grafts and various fixation methods (interference screws, staples, screw and washers) to reconstruct native anatomy. At our institution, we mostly employ combined Larson figure of eight and Muller popliteal bypass techniques, and these are described below.

The Larson figure of eight is used to reconstruct the popliteofibular ligament (PFL) and the LCL. As previously mentioned, the injured ligamentous structures in this area often have very frayed ends and are not amenable to direct repair so allograft or autograft tissue is used. Available donor tissue include the hamstrings (HS), tibialis anterior (TA), Achilles, or quadriceps; however, our preferred graft options are autograft hamstring including the semitendinosus and gracilis. Often, these autografts are needed for cruciate ligament reconstruction so semitendinosus allograft is most commonly selected. The larger diameter of the graft should be applied to the Muller popliteal bypass. For the Larson figure of eight, a length of at least 22–24 cm is required to allow for adequate fixation. The grafts are prepared on the back table using a #2 Fiberwire (Arthrex, Naples, Florida); however, any similarly robust suture placed in a whip-stitch technique would suffice.

While the graft is being prepared, the fibular tunnel for the Larson reconstruction is created. An anterior distal to posterior proximal tunnel is made through the thickest part of the fibular head, being very careful to retract the peroneal nerve out of the path of the drill bit. The tunnel is initially located with a guide wire over which we use a cannulated drill bit to finalize the preparation of our fibular tunnel. The tunnel sizes are chosen based on a sizing guide which measures the graft diameter. For semitendinosus and tibialis anterior, most tunnel sizes are 5 or 6 mm. For gracilis, the tunnel size is normally 4 or 4.5 mm.

The Muller popliteal bypass is then performed to reestablish the rotational control provided by the disrupted popliteus tendon. Using a second guide wire, we localize

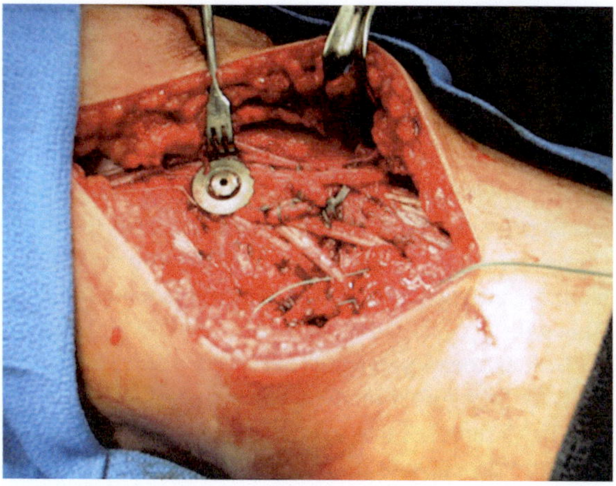

Fig. 4.4 Completed posterolateral corner reconstruction using a Muller popliteal bypass and Larson figure of eight. A large spiked washer was used for graft fixation (This image was published in Miller et al. [6], with permission)

our popliteus tunnel in the tibia with the intended trajectory being from Gerdy's tubercle to 1 cm medial and 1 cm inferior from the posterolateral aspect joint line of the tibia, i.e., the musculotendinous junction of the popliteus. Prior to placing this guide wire, the lateral head of the gastrocnemius and popliteus muscle is bluntly dissected off of the posterior tibia and retracted to protect the neurovascular structures. This is over-drilled with an appropriate-sized reamer. Next, the femoral insertion point for both grafts is located at the midpoint between the LCL insertion at the lateral epicondyle (which is usually palpable through the IT band) and the popliteus tendon insertion. A guide wire is placed to mark this location, but we do not yet drill this tunnel. Fluoroscopy is used to check the pin placement. One graft is then fed into the fibular tunnel with equal length kept on both sides. The two free ends of this graft are twisted and looped around the wire on lateral femoral epicondyle. The limb running from the anterior fibula to posterior to the guide wire re-creates the LCL. The second graft is fed through the tibia tunnel, around the posterolateral joint line, and looped around the wire as well. It is best to bring this graft initially anteriorly around the wire and then looping it counterclockwise. We use an 18-gauge Luque wire to facilitate this passage of the grafts through the tunnels. Additionally, we ensure that the graft limbs are deep to the IT band and biceps. At this point, the knee is taken through a full range of motion to assess for uniform graft tension as well as any restraints to flexion or extension. It is important that the wire is located at the isometric point as to not overtighten the joint and cause range of motion limitations postoperatively.

The original description of the Larson figure of eight involves creating a femoral socket in which the graft is placed and secured using a bioabsorbable screw +/− button fixation over the medial femoral cortex [14]. We usually choose to secure the two grafts with a large 6.5-mm cancellous screw and 17–22-mm spiked washer after twisting the Larson graft to form a figure of eight (Fig. 4.4). This is done to more accurately replicate the normal vector of these reconstructed soft tissue restraints. Once the guide wire location is confirmed to be isometric, the screw is placed approximately 1 cm proximal to the guide wire to account for the fact that the spiked washer will secure the grafts distal to where the screw is placed. For our tibial fixation, we use an interference screw backed up with a large staple at Gerdy's tubercle. The femoral-based screw and washer are tightened while the knee is held in 30° of flexion, and a slight valgus stress is applied to avoid any graft laxity. In our experience, these reconstructions do stretch out over time, so slightly over-tensioning the graft will ensure a stable PLC in the long term. Previously, we would place the knee in internal rotation, but we found that this inadvertently overtightened the posterolateral structures. In the situation where there is a native ligament or tendon stump remaining in the area where the graft is being placed, an attempt should be made to incorporate this tissue to augment the transplanted graft. This is often possible with the LCL where it can be sewn to the graft in a side-to-side fashion.

As mentioned previously, the drive-through sign can show if there is a capsular avulsion from either the femoral and tibial side, and our current PLC reconstruction includes a repair of this injury. We most often use suture anchors which can be used to secure the capsule back to the bone as well as repair the lateral meniscus at the same time (Fig. 4.5). This must be executed prior to securing the grafts or they will block your access to the anchor insertion sites. We feel that this is a simple step to augment the extra-articular reconstruction.

In our practice, the posterolateral structures are not secured until after the cruciates are reconstructed. Our rationale is that the central axis must be established first and then the PLC secured with the knee correctly positioned. If the patient has a disrupted ACL/PCL/PLC, this is the order that we follow: the ACL is fixed on the femur, the PCL is then fixed on the tibia, then the PLC is prepared and the grafts are passed. Then the PCL is fixed to restore the normal step off, followed by the ACL, and finally the PLC. Some surgeons reconstruct/repair the collaterals first and then the cruciates, and there is no universally accepted correct order.

Postoperatively, we place the patient in a hinged knee brace and 0–90° of motion is encouraged. If the PCL is also reconstructed at the same time, then our postoperative PCL protocol is followed.

4.3 Tips and Tricks

After reconstructing and repairing hundreds of PLC injuries, following are a few pearls that can make the case go more smoothly and safely.

- Be very thorough during your preoperative evaluation to fully appreciate all of the structures that may be damaged. This affects patient positioning and draping prior to making an incision.
- Do a diagnostic arthroscopy in order to assess intra-articular pathology before beginning to repair or reconstruct on the PLC. It is important to reconstruct or repair tissue in the appropriate sequence in order to not block your access. For example, secure the capsular avulsion back to the tibia or femur before repairing the torn biceps.
- Always have multiple allografts available in the operating room. You do not want to be stranded if you truncate your semitendinosus autograft during harvest or you have a diminutive gracilis.

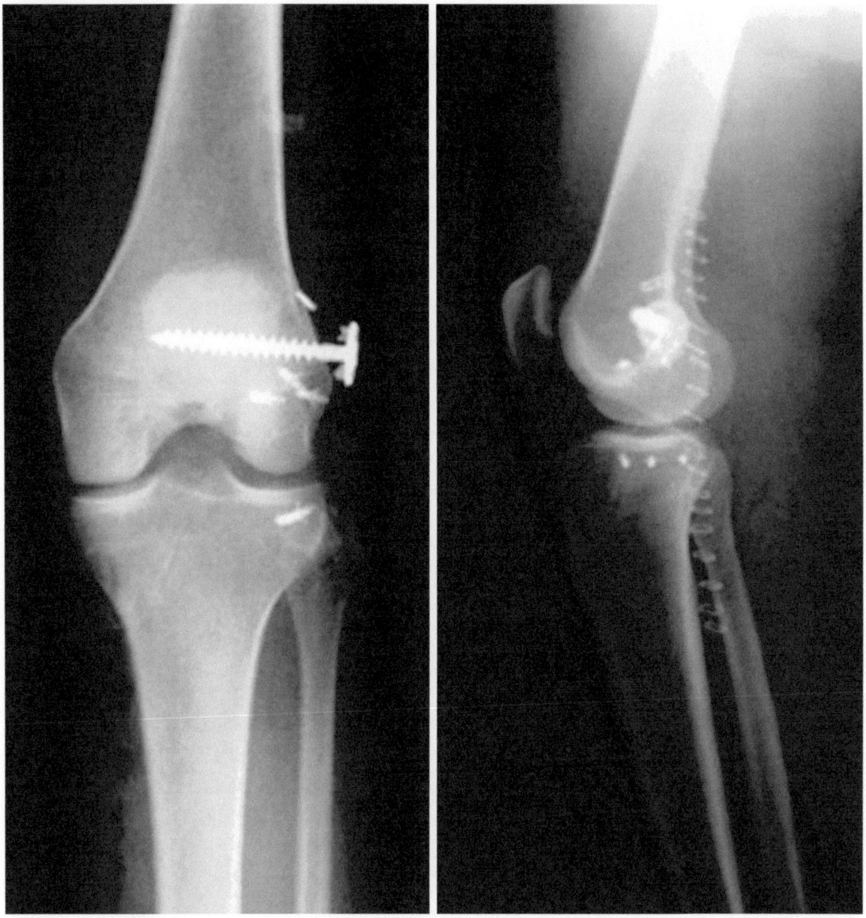

Fig. 4.5 AP and lateral radiographs of the completed posterolateral corner reconstruction. In this case, the lateral meniscus was avulsed off the tibia and was repaired with suture anchors. The popliteus tendon and the LCL were avulsed off their femoral insertions and also were anatomically repaired with suture anchors. Two free semitendinosis allografts were used for the posterolateral corner reconstruction and were fixed on the lateral femoral condyle. One graft was a Larson "Figure 8" graft across the fibular neck and another was a Muller popliteal bypass graft across the tibia. The patient also had a hamstring autograft ACL reconstruction

- Only use allografts of known origin. Check with your tissue bank to ensure that you are getting grafts from healthy, younger people versus people on dialysis. Allografts should have only low-dose irradiation at most. The strength and longevity of the reconstruction is very dependent on the tissue quality.
- Have multiple fixation methods at your disposal (suture anchors, screw and spiked washers, interference screws, small fragment set).
- While drilling the tibial tunnel for the Muller popliteal bypass, it is helpful to use the ACL guide to accurately guide the trajectory of the guide wire.

- Start the tibial tunnel on a flat point just distal and medial Gerdy's tubercle where there is not as much soft tissue to make it easier to find the tunnel later in the case.
- Confirm the location of your femoral tunnel using fluoroscopy.
- It is important to start the fibular tunnel more medial and inferior than one would think to avoid breaking off the fibular head.
- When using two grafts, use the longer one for the Larson. You need about 22–24 cm of graft and slightly less for the Muller.
- If the LCL is avulsed off of the femur, then the proximal part of the ligament can be integrated into the screw and washer construct. Confirm that the peroneal nerve is not also trapped.
- Postoperative rehab is a very important aspect of surgically addressing a PLC injury. We place the patient in a hinged knee brace for 6–8 weeks, start ROM exercises immediately, and keep the patient partial weight bearing. However, other surgically addressed injuries usually take precedence, such as if the PCL is reconstructed we will only allow early prone ROM.

4.4 Complications

It is important to have a lengthy discussion with the patient prior to undertaking a posterolateral corner reconstruction as this procedure, compared to other elective orthopedic procedures, is fraught with complications. It is difficult to accurately estimate the incidence of complications due to the multitude of various surgical techniques utilized. One the most dreaded complications is related to damage to the peroneal nerve. Based off of a literature review, it was noted that 12–17 % of acute PLC injuries have some level of peroneal nerve dysfunction either from the injury itself or from an intraoperative insult [15]. Surgical causes include excessive retraction, piercing the nerve while drilling the fibular tunnel, excessive tourniquet time causing a compressive and/or vascular insult, or passing suture around or through the nerve during wound closure. The popliteal artery is also at risk during the posterior knee dissection, especially during PCL fixation. If there was a prior vascular injury requiring repair or grafting, tourniquet use is discouraged due to the increased risk of thrombosis and damage to the graft [16]. Compartment syndrome is an equally as devastating complication and can occur from fluid extravasation from capsular rents caused at the time of injury. One of the arguments for delayed reconstruction of PLC injuries is that the risk of compartment syndrome is greatly reduced after the capsule heals; however, this risk can also be reduced by using gravity flow intraoperatively or by creating an egress arthrotomy which is often made by your standard open lateral approach to the knee.

Postoperatively, there is a risk that the repaired or reconstructed knee will continue to experience stability difficulties related to the initial ligamentous injury. As previously mentioned, Stannard observed a 9 % failure rate after reconstructed using the modified 2-tail technique [13]. There is always a concern for continued residual laxity related to tightening the grafts with the knee in varus or external rotation or to hardware failure or graft stretching. On the opposite end of the spectrum, restricted knee ROM postoperatively can be related to arthrofibrosis or to overtightening the grafts during tensioning. Securing PLC structures in internal rotation can produce such a predicament.

Even with preoperative and postoperative antibiotic administration, infection is documented in 0.3–12.5 % of knee reconstructions with higher risk with increased tourniquet time and with the creation of small skin bridges [17]. We have seen a few cases of late lateral femoral screw loosening which is painful for the patient, creates a palpable mass which irritates the IT band, and requires a return trip to the operating room for removal. Other less well studied but described complications include fibula fracture from tunnel placement and graft tensioning, painful hardware, deep venous thrombosis (DVT) and subsequent pulmonary emboli (PE), heterotopic ossification, reflex sympathetic dystrophy, persistent knee pain, and subsequent osteoarthritis.

4.5 Summary

Acutely addressing posterolateral corner injuries is preferred by many orthopedic surgeons because of the ability to more easily identify native structures and of outcome studies which show these patients have the best outcomes [8, 9]. There are many surgical techniques used to achieve translational and rotatory stability by repairing native structures and reconstructing others with soft tissue grafts. Here, we described our preferred method of the Larson figure of eight and Muller popliteal bypass and some tricks that we use to make this surgery successful.

References

1. LaPrade RF et al (2007) A prospective magnetic resonance imaging study of the incidence of posterolateral and multiple ligament injuries in acute knee injuries presenting with a hemarthrosis. Arthroscopy 23(12):1341–1347
2. Gardner MJ et al (2005) The incidence of soft tissue injury in operative tibial plateau fractures: a magnetic resonance imaging analysis of 103 patients. J Orthop Trauma 19(2):79–84
3. DeLee JC, Riley MB, Rockwood CA Jr (1983) Acute posterolateral rotatory instability of the knee. Am J Sports Med 11(4):199–207
4. LaPrade RF, Terry GC (1997) Injuries to the posterolateral aspect of the knee. Association of anatomic injury patterns with clinical instability. Am J Sports Med 25(4):433–438
5. Sekiya JK et al (2008) A clinically relevant assessment of posterior cruciate ligament and posterolateral corner injuries. Evaluation of isolated and combined deficiency. J Bone Joint Surg Am 90(8):1621–1627
6. Miller MD, Cole BJ, Cosgarea AJ, Sekiya JK (2008) Posterolateral corner reconstruction. In: Miller MD, Cole BJ, Cosgarea AJ, Sekiya JK (eds) Sports knee surgery. Saunders, Philadelphia, pp 361–376
7. LaPrade RF et al (2008) The reproducibility and repeatability of varus stress radiographs in the assessment of isolated fibular collateral ligament and grade-III posterolateral knee injuries. An in vitro biomechanical study. J Bone Joint Surg Am 90(10):2069–2076

8. Clancy WG Jr, Shepard MF, Cain EL Jr (2003) Posterior lateral corner reconstruction. Am J Orthop (Belle Mead NJ) 32(4):171–176
9. Veltri DM, Warren RF (1994) Operative treatment of posterolateral instability of the knee. Clin Sports Med 13(3):615–627
10. LaPrade RF (1997) Arthroscopic evaluation of the lateral compartment of knees with grade 3 posterolateral knee complex injuries. Am J Sports Med 25(5):596–602
11. LaPrade RF (2006) Posterolateral knee injuries: anatomy, evaluation, and treatment. Thieme, New York. xv, 238 p
12. Coobs BR et al (2007) Biomechanical analysis of an isolated fibular (lateral) collateral ligament reconstruction using an autogenous semitendinosus graft. Am J Sports Med 35(9):1521–1527
13. Stannard JP et al (2005) The posterolateral corner of the knee: repair versus reconstruction. Am J Sports Med 33(6):881–888
14. Fanelli GC, Larson RV (2002) Practical management of posterolateral instability of the knee. Arthroscopy 18(2 Suppl 1):1–8
15. Ranawat A et al (2008) Posterolateral corner injury of the knee: evaluation and management. J Am Acad Orthop Surg 16(9):506–518
16. Johnson ME, Foster L, DeLee JC (2008) Neurologic and vascular injuries associated with knee ligament injuries. Am J Sports Med 36(12):2448–2462
17. Lubowitz JH, Elson W, Guttmann D (2006) Complications in the treatment of medial and lateral sided injuries of the knee joint. Sports Med Arthrosc 14(1):51–55

Surgical Approach to Chronic Medial Injury

5

Alex G. Dukas and Thomas M. DeBerardino

Injury to the ligamentous medial knee has long been thought of as a simple medial collateral ligament (MCL) injury. Rather, the ligamentous medial knee is formed from a complex of structures that act synergistically to deliver static and dynamic stability. Injuries to the MCL complex are the most common ligamentous injuries to the knee and the majority of such can be treated successfully through nonoperative means [1, 2]. However, treatment modalities are continually debated, and operative measures are indicated in select patients.

The medial static stabilizers of the knee consist of the superficial medial collateral ligament (SMCL), deep medial collateral ligament (DMCL), and the posterior oblique ligament (POL). All three ligaments work concertedly to resist valgus and external rotation forces of the tibia relative to the femur [3]. The complex of ligaments also has a secondary stabilization role in anterior tibial translation [4, 5].

5.1 Biomechanics

To completely understand the function of the MCL complex, it is necessary to understand the anatomy (Fig. 5.1). The SMCL is the longest of the three with one femoral attachment and two tibial attachments. On the femur, it attaches just proximal and posterior to the medial epicondyle in the central sulcus of the medial epicondyle. The SMCL then courses distally to its first of two soft tissue attachments of the anterior arm of the semimembranosus tendon, then its second attachment approximately 5–7 cm below the joint line under the pes anserine bursa [6, 7]. Functionally, the SMCL is the primary restraint to valgus force. The SMCL has two divisions; the portion of the SMCL that spans the femur to proximal tibial

A.G. Dukas, MD, MA • T.M. DeBerardino, MD (✉)
Orthopaedic Surgery, UCONN Health Center,
263 Farmington Ave, MARB4, Farmington, CT 06032, USA
e-mail: dukas@uchc.edu; tdeber@uchc.edu, tdeberardino@live.com

R. Rossi, F. Margheritini (eds.), *Knee Ligament Injuries*,
DOI 10.1007/978-88-470-5513-1_5, © Springer Verlag Italia 2014

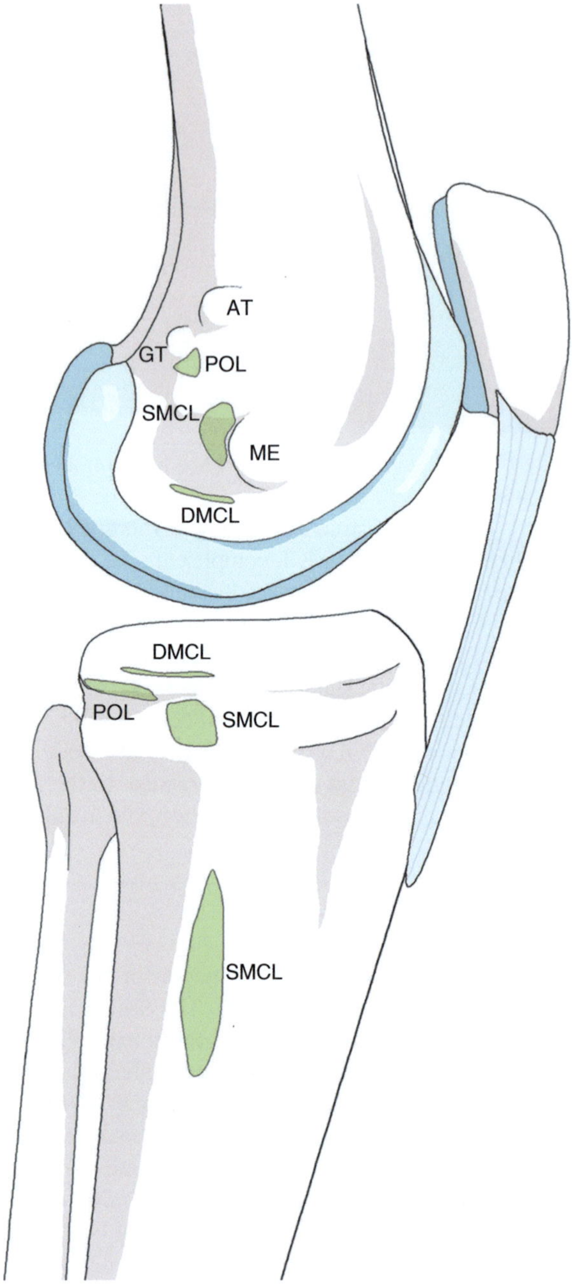

Fig. 5.1 Bony landmarks and ligament attachment sites. *GT* gastrocnemius tubercle, *AT* adductor tubercle, *POL* posterior oblique ligament, *SMCL* superficial medial collateral ligament, *ME* medial epicondyle, *DMCL* deep medial collateral ligament

attachment has a larger role in valgus stability while the distal portion plays a larger role in external rotation stability [8].

The DMCL is a short and broad capsular thickening that attaches firmly to the meniscus and just beyond each articular margin of the tibia and femur. It functions as a secondary restraint to valgus load at all flexion angles.

The POL is a triangular thickening of the joint capsule with a firm attachment to the posterior horn of the medial meniscus. It is composed of three different fascial expansions: the superficial, central, and capsular arms. The central arm is the main restraint component, which is reconstructed in the presented technique. Its femoral attachment is posterior to the SMCL lying just distal (2.9 mm) to the gastrocnemius tubercle, an osseous prominence coined by LaPrade et al., which is a very helpful intraoperative identification [6]. It can also be located distal and posterior to the adductor tubercle. The tibial attachment is anterior to the semimembranosus tendon with an expansion to the anterior portion of the semimembranosus tendon allowing the POL to be loose in flexion and taught in extension, especially with internal rotation.

5.2 Clinical Relevance

Clinically, the medial ligaments provide approximately 57 % of restraint to valgus stress at 5° flexion [9]. Increasing the flexion angle increases load bearing on these structures yielding up to 78 % of restraint at 25° [9]. When the distal portion of the SMCL is ruptured, studies have shown there to be just as much external rotation instability as found in posterior lateral corner disruptions [8].

There is however debate to the proper treatment of MCL complex injuries partly in due to the fact that the SMCL has served as a model for ligament healing in basic research. The SMCL has a large reserve for healing nonoperatively and is extrasynovial, unlike the ACL, which has poor healing reserve and typically requires surgical reconstruction. The healing process of the MCL has been well studied and consists of the inflammation phase (72 h), repair and regeneration phase (6 weeks), and the remodeling phase (can be present up to 1 year) [10].

Knee laxity is graded by medial joint opening with valgus force at 30°: 0 (normal), I (1–4 mm), II (5–9 mm), and III (10–15 mm). Grades I and II will have a hard endpoint, while grade II injuries will have a soft endpoint as the MCL is considered fully ruptured at this grade. Generally the preferred treatment for isolated acute MCL complex injury is nonoperative management. Grade I and II laxity require hinged bracing and guarded weight bearing initially followed by early range of motion. Nonoperative management has been shown to provide good patient-reported outcomes and even grade III type lesions go on to heal regularly with patients returning to full activity levels in 5–7 weeks time [7, 11–13].

However, studies have shown that grade III injuries often heal with less stability than the uninjured side [14]. Animal studies have demonstrated an increase in type III collagen scar following healing, resulting in increased laxity and only 70 % of initial strength [15–17]. Other studies have noted improved strength with surgical repair and improved results and strength with early nonoperative range of motion [2, 11, 18]. Propensity to heal is highly correlated with the location of the rupture with mid-substance tears reserving the most potential for healing, less so as one moves toward the bony attachments [19, 20].

However, isolated grade III injuries are rare. The majority of grade III lesions are associated with multiligamentous injury that requires operative treatment [10, 21].

5.3 Presentation

Patients with acute injuries usually present following a traumatic event with localized swelling and induration over some portion of the MCL location. Most low-grade sprains occur as noncontact injuries during a valgus and external rotation load. Complete MCL disruptions often result from a direct blow to the lateral leg. These pure valgus forces result in an isolated MCL injury. The addition of external rotation forces to the tibia expands the zone of injury to include the POL and/or the anterior cruciate ligament. As 78 % of all grade III injuries are multiligamentous, an audible pop and generalized intra-articular swelling might suggest anterior cruciate involvement [12]. Although often confounding in the acute patient, deep medial joint line tenderness can be indicative for medial meniscal injury.

Chronically MCL deficient patients will typically describe mostly side-to-side instability and pain. These patients tend to present after minor injury or activity aggravating their instability. The Swain test, described by Lonergan and Taylor, is a testing for chronic deficiency and rotatory instability [22]. Performed with the knee flexed to 90°, the tibia is then externally rotated. In this position the cruciate ligaments are lax while the collaterals are taught. Medial pain will often be present with chronic laxity or inadequate ligament healing. While in this position, one can perform anteromedial drawer test to evaluate POL integrity [5]. Valgus gapping at 30° flexion will evaluate SMCL stability. Valgus gapping with the knee in full extension is more indicative of a combined SMCL and POL injury [23]. Of note, patients with a POL injury may also exhibit a positive Dial test, as anterior rotatory instability due to deficient POL will confound this test [5]. All grade III tears should undergo examination for concomitant cruciate injury, as mentioned above most are not isolated MCL injuries. Any evidence of genu valgum should be evaluated and treated before attempts are made to reconstruct medial ligaments.

Care should be taken to obtain high-quality radiographs on all patients. In addition to evaluation of fractures, avulsions, and loose bodies, radiographs should be obtained to delineate previous hardware and tunnel placement, osteophyte formation mechanical alignment, and lateral capsular signs (Segond's fracture); Pellegrini-Stieda lesions are specific for chronic MCL lesions. Stress views to evaluate gapping, and physeal injuries in adolescents should also be obtained.

MRI can be most useful when coupled with the physical exam to delineate the location of MCL tears, meniscal tears, cartilage lesions, and associated cruciate lesions.

5.4 Surgical Indications and Contraindications

While indications for surgical reconstruction of MCL complex injuries still remain highly debated, the set of indications the senior author follow are listed in Table 5.1.

Table 5.1 Surgical indications and contraindications

Indications	Bony avulsion injury Chronic instability Continued instability beyond 6 weeks of nonoperative management Failed ACL repair with medial instability
Contraindications	Isolated grade I or II injuries Skin disruption or breakdown over medial skin

5.5 Technique

In a subset of the acutely injured, operative repair of the effected medial ligaments is indicated. In patients who are initially treated by nonoperative means but continue to show valgus instability and are clinically symptomatic, reconstruction is indicated. It has been the experience of the senior author that optimal function of the MCL complex deficient patient is restored through reconstruction that reestablishes the patient's native anatomy. The technique of the senior author involves a reconstruction of the proximal and distal divisions of the SMCL and POL using two separate grafts.

The patient is placed supine on the surgical bed. General anesthesia is used. A thigh tourniquet is applied to the operative leg. The foot of the bed is flexed maximally with enough room behind the flexed knee to allow a fist to be placed in times when manipulation is required during the procedure. Two rolled sheets placed under the pad of the bed prevent hyperextension at the hip. The contralateral lower extremity is safely cradled in a well-type leg holder with the fibular head well padded. The nonoperative leg is also fixed with the knee and hip slightly flexed and abducted (Fig. 5.2).

After anesthesia is induced the operative knee undergoes a thorough examination for range of motion and ligamentous stability. After the patient is sterilely prepped and draped, a time-out is performed, and prophylactic antibiotics are administered.

Landmarks of the medial knee are identified via palpation and subsequently noted (refer to figure). An anteromedial incision initiating approximately half the distance to the adductor tubercle from the medial border of the patella, over the vastus medialis oblique running to the anteromedial portion of the tibia roughly 8 cm distal to the joint line. The superficial sartorial fascia is incised and the tendons of the semitendinosus and gracilis are identified. Deep to the pes anserine bursa is the distal portion of the SMCL, which is approximately 6 cm distal to the joint line. At this time a graft fixation tunnel is created by firstly placing an eyelet passing pin through the posterior portion of the distal SMCL attachment site transversely through the tibia aimed toward the fibular head. Care is then taken to pass a 7 mm reamer to a depth of 25 mm to form the reconstruction tunnel. LaPrade et al. have suggested placing the tunnel at the posterior portion of the distal attachment site as the more anterior position may result in graft failure [8].

Next focus is turned to the tibial POL portion of the reconstruction. Careful dissection through a small incision in the sartorial fascia at the anterior edge of the

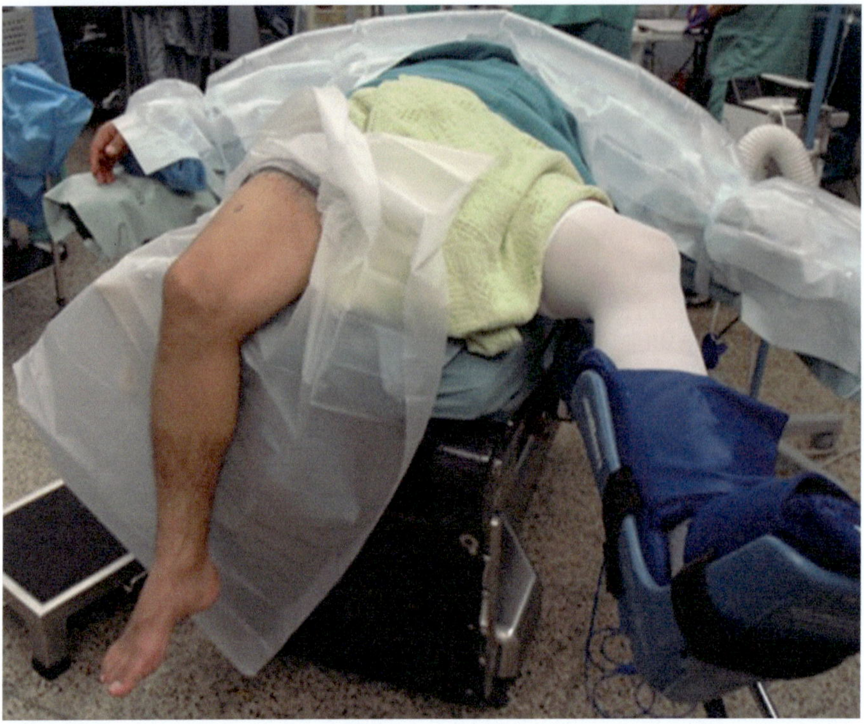

Fig. 5.2 Patient position and setup before sterile draping

semimembranosus tendon is made to identify the POL tibial attachment just anterior to the direct arm of the semimembranosus tendon. When confirmation of the tibial attachment has been made, sharp dissection is used to clear soft tissue to the bone. Just as with the SMCL tibial attachment, an eyelet pin is passed transversely through the tibia this time aiming anteriorly toward Gerdy's tubercle, followed by a 7 mm reamer to a depth of 25 mm to form the graft tunnel.

Attention is next focused on the femoral attachments of the SMCL and POL. Identify the posterior edge of the VMO and following the adductor magnus tendon down to its insertion is the landmark used to identify both the femoral origins of the SMCL and POL. After locating the VMO insertion, advance anteriorly approximately 5 mm to locate the SMCL origin, slightly proximal and posterior to the medial epicondyle. A standard guide pin is placed, but not overreamed with a 7 mm cannulated drill until the correct identification of the POL is made. If the reconstruction is in the setting of a cruciate rupture and repair or the patient has had a previous cruciate repair, care must be taken to have a more proximal trajectory as to avoid PCL tunnels.

The femoral attachment of the POL is posterior and distal to the site of attachment of the adductor magnus. The POL femoral attachment is 7.7 mm distal and 2.9 mm anterior to the gastrocnemius tubercle. Identification is made of the central arm portion of the POL by visualization of the vertical fibers in the joint capsular thickening. Once the POL origin is identified, an eyelet passing pin is placed in a parallel fashion and then a 7 mm cannulated reamer forms a 25 mm deep socket. The SMCL socket is formed in a similar fashion.

At this point, attention is turned toward the soft tissue graft preparation. Autograft hamstring (semitendinosus) or similar allograft hamstring is routinely used. Graft length is prepared by making the SMCL graft 16 cm in length and the POL graft 12 cm. These lengths fit the majority of reconstructions, but adjustments in size may be needed for patients at the extremes of size. The grafts are prepped by placing Fiberwire (Arthrex Naples, Fl) sutures in a Krakow configuration at both ends of each graft for fixation.

Using a passing suture the POL graft is passed into its femoral tunnel. Adequate depth recession into the tunnel is checked (about 2 cm). This process is repeated for the SMCL graft. Each graft is then secured with a biocomposite cannulated screw (Arthrex, Naples, FL) while ensuring the graft is in anatomical position as the screw position is finalized. Each graft is trialed under simple tension by hand to ensure the fixation screw has adequate purchase.

At this time, if there are other ligamentous repairs or reconstructions being performed at the time of procedure, the grafts are secured in their respective tunnels before moving on to distal fixation of the medial-sided structures.

The distal portions of each graft are then passed under the intact retinaculum fascia to their distally located and respective tunnels. Fiberwire passing sutures are then put into position via passing pins and subsequently used to pass the graft sutures into their respective tunnels. The SMCL graft is tensioned first with the knee in 20° of flexion with a slight varus force on the knee. A cannulated screw (Biotenodesis screw, Arthrex, Naples, FL) is used to secure the graft in its tunnel. The reconstructed SMCL is observed and inspected during range of motion to ensure there is no obvious over-tension or restriction of movement.

The leg is then pulled into full extension; the POL graft is tensioned and secured with a cannulated screw (Biotenodesis screw, Arthrex, Naples, FL). Again the knee is observed and inspected through range of motion ensuring there is no sign of over-tensioning or resistance to flexion-extension. The POL should be taunt in extension and slack in flexion as it is in its natural state. Valgus force is applied to the knee in 0° and 20° of flexion to inspect for any instability and ensure graft utility.

At this stage of the reconstruction, the SMCL and POL have been secured to their anatomic bony insertions; however, the native SMCL has a soft tissue attachment to the anterior portion of the semimembranosus tendon. To address this a suture anchor is placed 12 mm distal to the joint line and under and in line with the SMCL. The author uses a biocomposite soft tissue anchor (Arthrex, Naples, FL). Once the anchor is secured, the suture tails are passed through the native remnant and SMCL graft recreating the proximal soft tissue connection of the native SMCL. Again the grafts are tensioned as the knee is cycled through a range of motion to ensure the anatomic reconstruction is successful. The superficial retinaculum is then closed over the reconstruction (refer to Fig. 5.3).

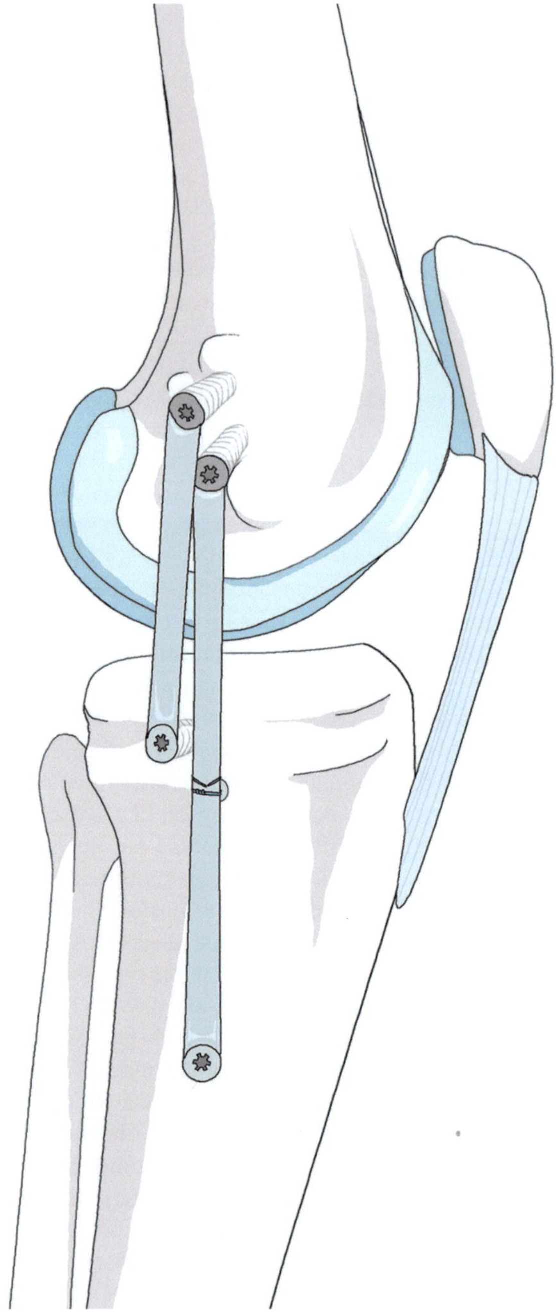

Fig. 5.3 Schematic of anatomic superficial medial collateral and posterior oblique ligament reconstruction

5.6 Postoperative Course

After anatomic MCL complex reconstruction has been performed, postoperative therapy is aimed at preventing quadriceps atrophy and intra-articular adhesion formation. Within the first week postoperatively, the patient begins physical therapy with limited range of motion. The patient is kept non-weight bearing for the first 6 weeks. Physical therapy during the initial 6 weeks focuses on closed chain exercises and quadriceps strengthening. After the initial 6 weeks, progression to full weight bearing is allowed and reestablishing normal range of motion is the goal. During this initial time period, there are multiple interval scheduled follow-up office visits to ensure successful postoperative course and patient adherence.

References

1. Lind M, Jakobsen BW, Lund B, Hansen MS, Abdallah O, Christiansen SE (2009) Anatomical reconstruction of the medial collateral ligament and posteromedial corner of the knee in patients with chronic medial collateral ligament instability. Am J Sports Med 37:1116–1122
2. Liu X, Feng H, Zhang H et al (2013) Surgical treatment of subacute and chronic valgus instability in multiligament-injured knees with superficial medial collateral ligament reconstruction using Achilles allografts: a quantitative analysis with a minimum 2-year follow-up. Am J Sports Med 41:1044–1050
3. Azar FM (2006) Evaluation and treatment of chronic medial collateral ligament injuries of the knee. Sports Med Arthrosc 14:84–90
4. Marchant MH Jr, Tibor LM, Sekiya JK, Hardaker WT Jr, Garrett WE Jr, Taylor DC (2011) Management of medial-sided knee injuries, part 1: medial collateral ligament. Am J Sports Med 39:1102–1113
5. Tibor LM, Marchant MH Jr, Taylor DC, Hardaker WT Jr, Garrett WE Jr, Sekiya JK (2011) Management of medial-sided knee injuries, part 2: posteromedial corner. Am J Sports Med 39:1332–1340
6. LaPrade RF, Engebretsen AH, Ly TV, Johansen S, Wentorf FA, Engebretsen L (2007) The anatomy of the medial part of the knee. J Bone Joint Surg Am 89:2000–2010
7. Phisitkul P, James SL, Wolf BR, Amendola A (2006) MCL injuries of the knee: current concepts review. Iowa Orthop J 26:77–90
8. Coobs BR, Wijdicks CA, Armitage BM et al (2010) An in vitro analysis of an anatomical medial knee reconstruction. Am J Sports Med 38:339–347
9. Grood ES, Noyes FR, Butler DL, Suntay WJ (1981) Ligamentous and capsular restraints preventing straight medial and lateral laxity in intact human cadaver knees. J Bone Joint Surg Am 63:1257–1269
10. Thomas M, DeBerardino SAW (2010) Management of patients with combined ACL and medial collateral ligament insufficiency. In: Bach BR, Provencher MT (eds) ACL surgery: how to get it right the first time and what to do if it fails. SLACK, Thorofare, NJ, pp 281–286
11. Canata GL, Chiey A, Leoni T (2012) Surgical technique: does mini-invasive medial collateral ligament and posterior oblique ligament repair restore knee stability in combined chronic medial and ACL injuries? Clin Orthop Relat Res 470:791–797
12. Sims WF, Jacobson KE (2004) The posteromedial corner of the knee: medial-sided injury patterns revisited. Am J Sports Med 32:337–345

13. Bauer KL, Stannard JP (2013) Surgical approach to the posteromedial corner: indications, technique, outcomes. Curr Rev Musculoskelet Med 6:124–131
14. Abramowitch SD, Yagi M, Tsuda E, Woo SL (2003) The healing medial collateral ligament following a combined anterior cruciate and medial collateral ligament injury–a biomechanical study in a goat model. J Orthop Res 21:1124–1130
15. Frank C, Woo SL, Amiel D, Harwood F, Gomez M, Akeson W (1983) Medial collateral ligament healing. A multidisciplinary assessment in rabbits. Am J Sports Med 11:379–389
16. Frank C, Amiel D, Woo SL, Akeson W (1985) Normal ligament properties and ligament healing. Clin Orthop Relat Res 196:15–25
17. Frank CB, Loitz BJ, Shrive NG (1995) Injury location affects ligament healing. A morphologic and mechanical study of the healing rabbit medial collateral ligament. Acta Orthop Scand 66:455–462
18. Osti L, Papalia R, Del Buono A, Merlo F, Denaro V, Maffulli N (2010) Simultaneous surgical management of chronic grade-2 valgus instability of the knee and anterior cruciate ligament deficiency in athletes. Knee Surg Sports Traumatol Arthrosc 18:312–316
19. Hughston JC, Eilers AF (1973) The role of the posterior oblique ligament in repairs of acute medial (collateral) ligament tears of the knee. J Bone Joint Surg Am 55:923–940
20. Woo SL, Chan SS, Yamaji T (1997) Biomechanics of knee ligament healing, repair and reconstruction. J Biomech 30:431–439
21. Zaffagnini S, Bignozzi S, Martelli S, Lopomo N, Marcacci M (2007) Does ACL reconstruction restore knee stability in combined lesions?: an in vivo study. Clin Orthop Relat Res 454:95–99
22. Lonergan K, Taylor D (2002) Medial collateral ligament injuries of the knee: an evolution of surgical reconstruction. Tech Knee Surg 1(2):137–145
23. Stannard JP (2010) Medial and posteromedial instability of the knee: evaluation, treatment, and results. Sports Med Arthrosc 18:263–268

Chronic Posteromedial Instability: Reconstruction Techniques

6

Davide E. Bonasia, Simone Spolaore, Corrado Bertolo, and Roberto Rossi

6.1 Introduction

Injuries to the medial collateral ligament (MCL) and posteromedial corner (PMC) of the knee are relatively common. The incidence of MCL/PMC lesions has been reported to be 0.24 per 1,000 people in the United States every year [1]. These lesions can be isolated or combined with other ligamentous injuries. Understanding the complicated relationship between anatomic structures and their unique biomechanical function is essential in diagnosing and treating these injuries. The vast majority of medial knee injuries heal with conservative treatment. However, some medial knee injuries result in chronic instability and functional limitations. The high reparative potential of the MCL with conservative treatment and the complications (mainly knee stiffness) associated with surgical treatment are at the base of the controversies regarding the treatment of MCL/PMC injuries in the acute setting. Although surgery is the only option in treating chronic medial instability, no decision algorithms are available and a wide variety of surgical techniques have been described regarding this topic.

The aim of this chapter is to describe the most commonly used PMC reconstruction techniques. Technical notes and literature results are also presented. Elements of anatomy and biomechanics specifically related to the medial and posteromedial

D.E. Bonasia (✉)
Department of Orthopaedics and Traumatology,
Azienda ospedaliera Città della Salute e della Scienza,
Presidio ospedaliero CTO, Via Lamarmora 26, Torino 10128, Italy
e-mail: davidebonasia@virgilio.it

S. Spolaore • C. Bertolo
Department of Orthopaedics and Traumatology,
Università degli Studi di Torino, Via Verdi 8, Torino 10124, Italy
e-mail: simo.spola@libero.it; corrado.bertolo@gmail.com

R. Rossi
Department of Orthopaedics and Traumatology,
Mauriziano "Umberto I" Hospital, Largo Turati 62, Torino 10128, Italy
e-mail: rossir@fastwebnet.it

R. Rossi, F. Margheritini (eds.), *Knee Ligament Injuries*,
DOI 10.1007/978-88-470-5513-1_6, © Springer Verlag Italia 2014

aspect of the knee are described, in order to better understand the different surgical procedures.

6.2 Anatomy and Biomechanics

For the MCL anatomy we refer to the specific chapters of this volume. The PMC includes the structures lying from the posterior border of the longitudinal fibers of the superficial MCL (sMCL) to the medial border of the posterior cruciate ligament (Fig. 6.1). These include the semimembranosus expansions, the posteromedial horn of the meniscus, the posterior oblique ligament (POL), the posteromedial capsule, and also the popliteal oblique ligament. POL is one of the most misunderstood structures of the medial aspect of the knee. It consists in three arms and three fascial attachments: superficial, central (tibial), and capsular. The primary component is the central arm, which attaches directly to the posterior meniscus and the joint capsule [2]. Mueller previously described the PMC as the "semimembranosus corner" as this structure has a significant functional contribution to the dynamic stability of the PMC [3]. The attachment of the semimembranosus muscle to the tibia acts as a dynamic stabilizer of the PMC [4]. In order to understand the biomechanical function of the structures of the PMC, one must also know the role of the MCL complex. Biomechanically, the MCL represents the main restraint to valgus forces and a secondary restraint to external/internal rotation and posterior translation of the tibia. The contribution of the sMCL to internal rotation stability increases beyond 30° of knee flexion when the posteromedial capsule is slackened. Instead, the posteromedial capsule is in tension and provides some stability to valgus forces, posterior tibial translation, and internal rotation only with the knee extended. The POL provides secondary stability to tibial internal and external rotation at early knee flexion as well as posterior stability to the tibia in full extension. The role of the POL

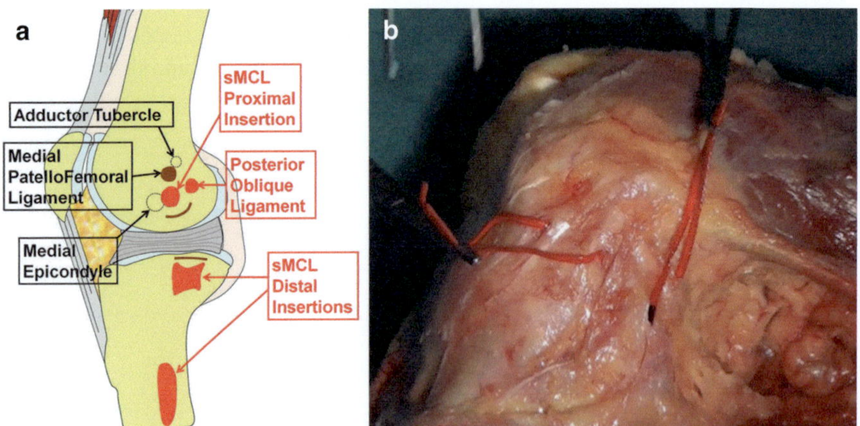

Fig. 6.1 (**a**) Medial view of the knee: attachment sites (Redrawn from Bonasia et al. [17]). (**b**) Medial aspect of the knee showing the MCL (*left loop*) and the POL (*right loop*)

becomes even more important in the setting of MCL deficiency in both valgus and rotational stability [5–7].

6.3 Diagnosis

In the diagnosis of MCL lesions, the authors prefer the Fetto and Marshall classification. This classification divides medial-sided knee injuries into grade 1 (no valgus laxity), grade 2 (valgus laxity at 30° of flexion), and grade 3 (valgus laxity at 0° and 30°) [8]. The stability of the knee is then tested in all planes in order to evaluate anteroposterior, lateral, and rotational instability.

By definition, patients with medial-sided injuries have increased laxity with valgus stress. The examiner applies a valgus stress to the knee at both 0° and 30° of flexion. For isolated sMCL injuries, the greatest joint space opening occurs with the knee in 30° of flexion [9]. Joint space opening with the knee fully extended indicates an injury to the capsule, the POL, or both. Grade III MCL injuries are frequently associated with injury to another ligament (mostly the ACL) [2].

Other physical examination maneuvers combine rotation with various amounts of knee flexion in an attempt to discriminate between MCL and MCL/PMC injuries. One of the most common involves a valgus stress to the knee in 30° of flexion with the foot externally rotated [2]. The presence of anteromedial rotary instability (AMRI) is indicative of PMC injury. AMRI is detected by performing the anterior drawer test with the tibia both in neutral and in external rotation. Increased translation with the tibia in external rotation is indicative of AMRI [10, 11]. Increased external rotation and AMRI indicate injury to the PMC and possibly to the ACL as well.

Weight-bearing radiographs of the knee are obtained in anteroposterior and lateral views. If valgus malalignment is present, a weight-bearing long-leg radiograph is obtained. MRI is helpful in diagnosing associated bone and soft tissue injuries (anterior and posterior cruciate ligaments, posterolateral corner, and menisci) as well as determining the location and extent of medial/posteromedial ligamentous injuries. However, it has been shown that MRI tends to overestimate injury to ligamentous structures [12].

6.4 Indications

In the acute setting (<3 weeks), the treatment of grade I–II injuries is mostly conservative [13, 14], but significant controversies exist regarding the treatment of grade III lesions, both isolated and combined with other ligamentous injuries [15, 16].

On the other hand, in the chronic (>6 weeks) medial/posteromedial instability setting, the conservative treatment option can be excluded. However, controversies exist regarding the most reliable surgical technique. In addition, the limb alignment is a crucial predicting factor and needs to be carefully evaluated. In case of varus or neutral alignment, only soft tissue procedures addressing the medial instability should be performed. In case of severe valgus, a distal femoral varus osteotomy with or without soft tissue procedures should to be considered.

In case of combined PMC and ACL instability, ACL reconstruction is performed and the knee is evaluated intraoperatively for medial laxity. If the knee shows at full extension a medial opening greater than 4 mm compared to the contralateral side, capsular procedures or MCL reconstruction can be considered [17]. This has to be carefully considered while planning the surgery in order to leave adequate graft options for PMC reconstruction after the ACL procedure. In these cases, the authors recommend patellar tendon or allograft ACL reconstruction, in order to preserve the hamstrings for the PMC procedures. Alternatively, allografts can be used for PMC reconstruction.

In case of multiligament knee injuries [18, 19], these are generally treated acutely, but in some cases (i.e., polytrauma), the procedure can be delayed, respecting the damage control principles. In case of chronic multiligament knee injuries in young patients, the authors' approach is to treat all torn ligaments with allograft reconstruction procedures at the same time. Alternatively, only ACL reconstruction can be delayed.

Many techniques have been described for the treatment of medial and posteromedial ligamentous injuries of the knee, either with allograft or autograft. These can be divided in capsular procedures and reconstruction techniques.

6.5 Capsular Procedures

In these procedures the lax medial/posteromedial structures are re-tensioned but not reconstructed. The surgical approach is as previously described in specific chapters of this volume.

6.5.1 Re-tensioning of the Posteromedial Structures

The goal of this technique is to create increased distance between the origin and insertion of the lax medial/posteromedial structures. This is done by attaching the lax segments of the tendon/ligament to an adjacent intact structure. Therefore, this procedure is indicated when some medial or posteromedial structures are intact. There are no strict rules regarding the re-tension of lax structures, because this depends on the patient's injury pattern. However, different structures need to be visualized and probed for tension, and these include the sMCL, the posteromedial capsule, the medial meniscus attachments, the POL, and the capsular arm of the semimembranosus tendon.

The sartorius fascia is incised longitudinally and care is taken to avoid injury to the saphenous nerve. The whole MCL is probed (proximal and distal attachments as well as mid-substance). Once the posteromedial capsule is visualized and palpated for laxity, a longitudinal arthrotomy is performed posterior to the MCL. The capsular arm of the semimembranosus is identified and probed for tension. The POL and the meniscotibial attachments are evaluated. Every lax structure is armed and sutured to an intact adjacent ligament/tendon or back to the bone with transosseous sutures. Multiple reinforcing sutures can be placed across the POL and MCL.

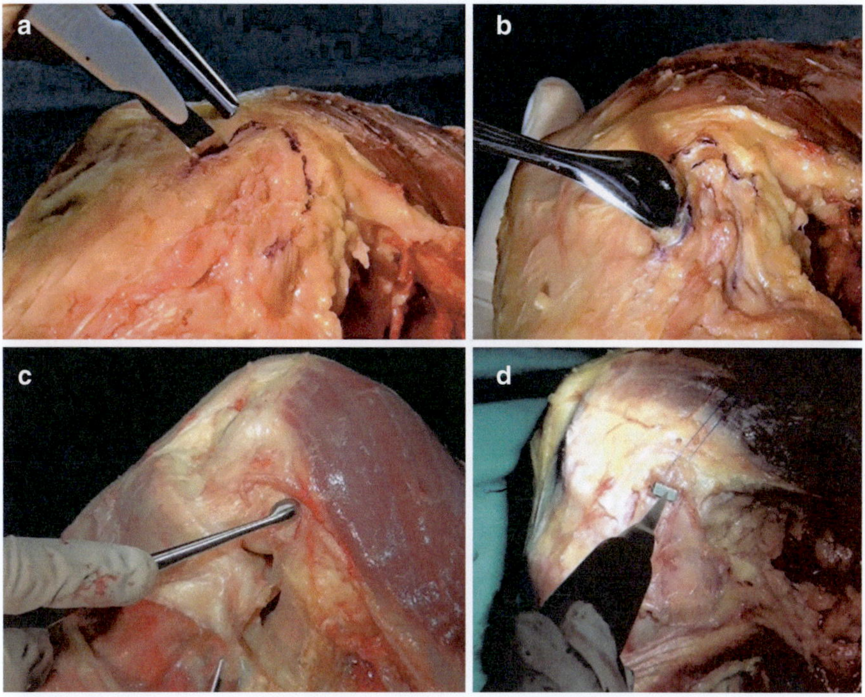

Fig. 6.2 En masse elevation. (**a**, **b**) The structures at the weakest attachment (in this specimen, the femoral attachment) are released as an entire tendon/ligament unit (en masse). (**c**) The bone around the isometric point is "roughed-up" until a good bleeding is achieved. (**d**) Fixation is achieved with staples or suture anchors

6.5.2 En Masse Elevation

This procedure is indicated when a generalized laxity of the medial/posteromedial structures is present. A medial hockey-stick incision is preferred, from the pes anserinus to the posterior portion of the medial femoral epicondyle. The weakest attachment (femoral or tibial) of the medial/posteromedial complex should be identified. The structures at the weakest attachment must be released as an entire tendon/ligament unit (en masse) and not as individual tendons or ligaments, in order to preserve their integrity and vascularity (Fig. 6.2). This unit must be strongly armed with sutures, re-tensioned, and fixed back to the bone. Reattachment to the bone is performed anteriorly and inferiorly if the tibial insertion is lax or posteriorly and superiorly in case of femoral insertion laxity. The bone around the isometric point is "roughed-up" until good bleeding is achieved. Fixation can be achieved with staples or suture anchors [20, 21]. As in the acute MCL repair, care must be taken to preserve the isometricity, mostly when a proximal en masse elevation is performed, in order to reduce the risk of postoperative stiffness.

6.6 Reconstruction Techniques

6.6.1 Kim's Technique

A curvilinear incision is placed from the medial femoral epicondyle to the pes anserinus. The sartorius and gracilis tendons are retracted medially. The semitendinosus is harvested, preserving the tibial attachment. The proximal end of the tendon is armed with a n°2 nonabsorbable suture. A 1.6 mm K wire is placed on the postero-superior border of the medial femoral epicondyle. The semitendinosus tendon is looped around the wire, and isometricity (<2 mm migration) is tested through a full range of motion. A 6.5 mm cancellous screw and an 18 mm diameter soft tissue washer are placed through a hole. The screw hole is drilled 9 mm (the radius of the washer) proximal to the isometric point. Decortication is performed around the drill hole. After manual tensioning of the graft, the screw is tightened with the knee in 30° of flexion and varus stress (Fig. 6.3). Dissection of the direct head of the semimembranous tendon is performed. The free end of the graft is pulled under the direct head of the semimembranosus tendon and sutured to it at 30° of knee flexion [22].

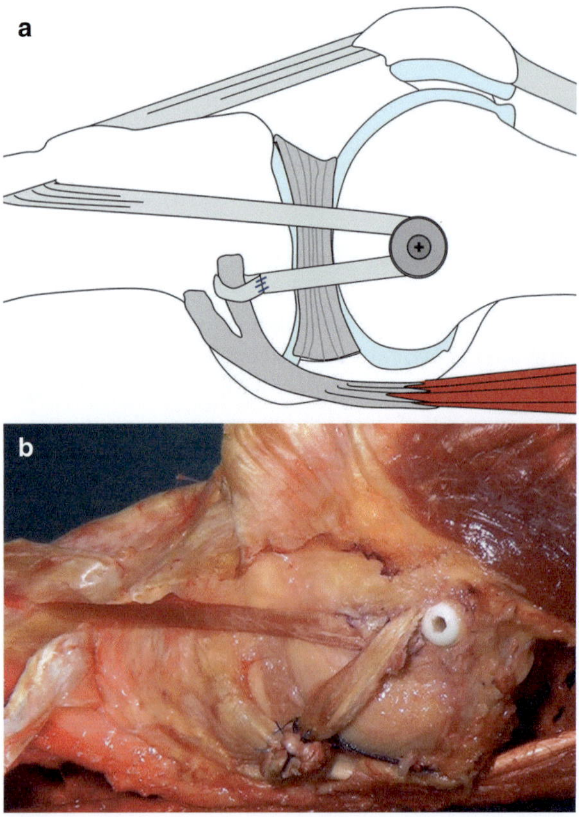

Fig. 6.3 (**a**) Kim's technique (see text) (Redrawn from Bonasia et al. [17]). (**b**) Specimen showing the reconstruction (in this case with an interference screw, instead of screw and washer)

6.6.2 Stannard's Technique

In Stannard's modification of Kim's technique, the free end of the semitendinosus is passed under the direct head of the semimembranosus tendon and sutured to the intact insertion of the semitendinosus itself on the tibia (Fig. 6.4). The graft is tensioned with the knee in approximately 40° of flexion and a slight varus stress [23].

6.6.3 Lind's Technique

Incision, semitendinosus harvesting, and isometricity evaluation are as described by Kim. A tunnel of the same size of the double-looped tendon is drilled at the isometric point on the femur. The tendon loop is then armed with a baseball suture, passed into the tunnel, and fixed with an interference screw (same diameter as the tunnel or 1 mm bigger according to the bone quality). This is performed with the knee at 10° of flexion and neutral rotation. A tibial tunnel (same size of the graft) is then drilled to the posterior corner of the medial tibial condyle from anterior to posterior. The drill hole is aimed to exit 10 mm below the tibial plateau, posterior and lateral to the semimembranosus insertion. The free end of the graft is passed through the

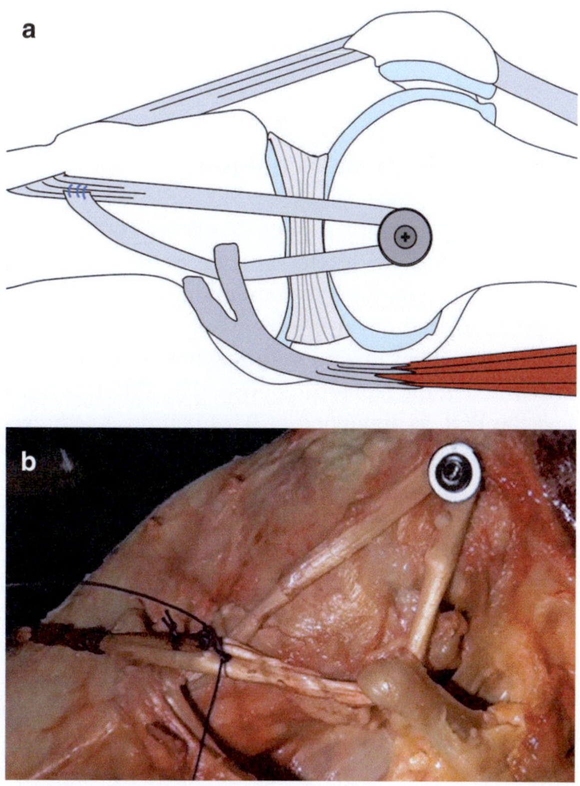

Fig. 6.4 (**a**) Stannard's modification of Kim's technique (see text) (Redrawn from Bonasia et al. [17]). (**b**) Specimen showing the reconstruction

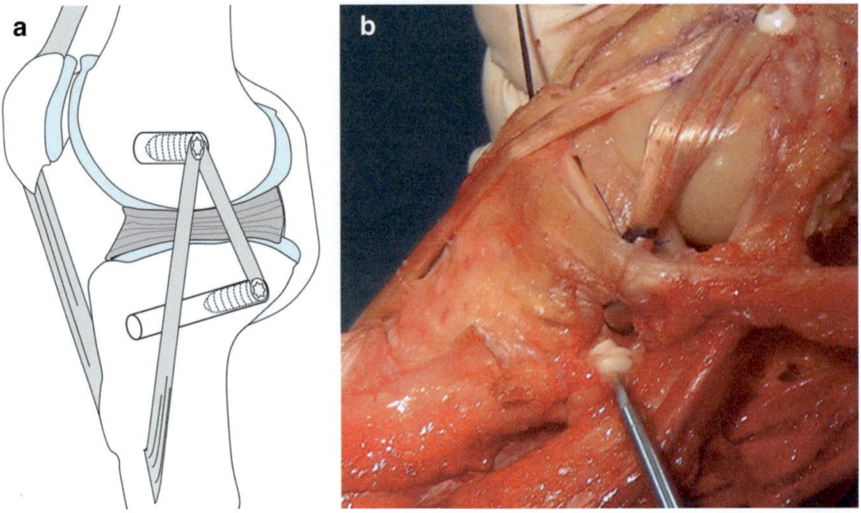

Fig. 6.5 (**a**) Lind's technique (see text) (Redrawn from Bonasia et al. [17]). (**b**) Specimen showing the reconstruction

posterior tibial tunnel opening and fixed here with an interference screw (same diameter as the tunnel) to reconstruct the POL (Fig. 6.5). This is tightened at 60° of flexion and neutral rotation [24].

6.6.4 Coobs et al. Technique

This technique entails a reconstruction of both sMCL and POL, through a single medial incision, with two separate grafts and four different tunnels (Fig. 6.6). Allografts or gracilis and semitendinosus autografts can be used. The anatomy of proximal and distal insertions of both bundles needs to be known (Fig. 6.1). Isometricity is evaluated with K wires for both bundles. Correctly sized tunnels are drilled at the isometric points. The sMCL is tightened at 30° of knee flexion and the POL is tightened at 0°. Fixation is achieved with interference screws [25, 26].

6.6.5 Borden's Technique

With a 2-incision approach, a guide pin is drilled into the medial epicondyle. Next, a n°2 suture is looped over the guide pin and retrieved (along the MCL) from the tibial incision (Fig. 6.7). Isometricity is tested by holding the suture at the anterior aspect of the MCL tibial insertion and moving the knee through a full range of motion. Another guide pin is placed into the tibia at this isometric point. Isometricity can be tested again with a suture looped around both guide pins

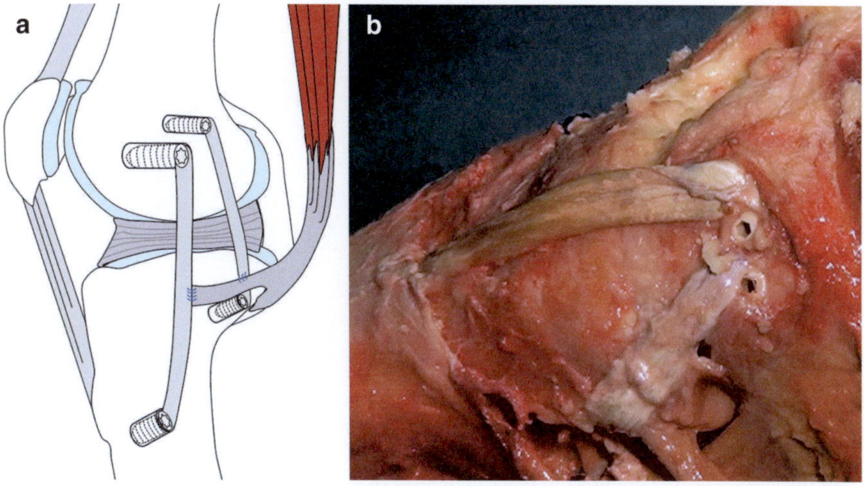

Fig. 6.6 (**a**) Coobs et al. technique (see text) (Redrawn from Bonasia et al. [17]). (**b**) Specimen showing the reconstruction

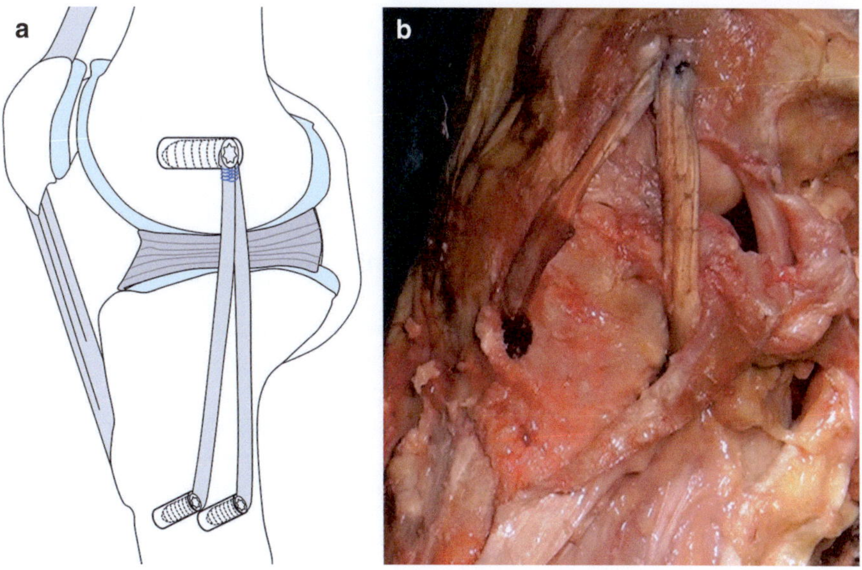

Fig. 6.7 (**a**) Borden's technique (see text) (Redrawn from Bonasia et al. [17]). (**b**) Specimen showing the reconstruction

(Fig. 6.8). The hamstring tendons are then retracted posteromedially. The isometric point for the posterior tibial tunnel is then determined in a similar fashion. A second pin is placed. A tibialis anterior tendon allograft is prepared in a double-bundle loop. Alternatively, an autologous semitendinosus tendon can be used.

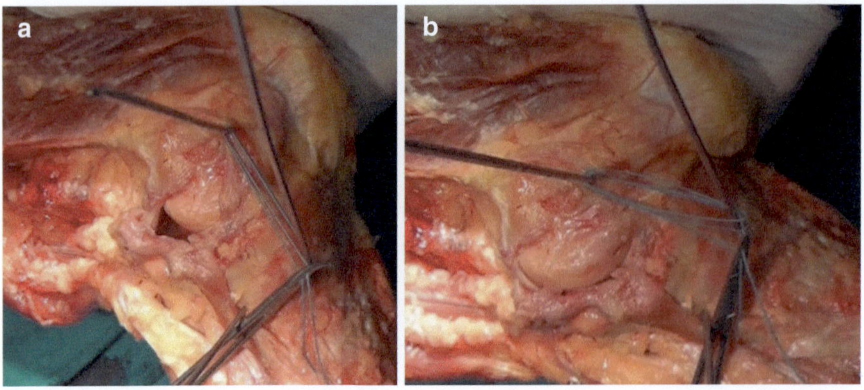

Fig. 6.8 Technique to find the isometric points. In this case, 2 K wires are positioned at the presumptive isometric points. A suture is then looped around the K wires and held with a Kelly clamp, while the knee is moved through full range of motion. In this case the points are not isometric: note the suture tight in flexion (**a**) and slack in extension (**b**)

One 30 mm long femoral tunnel and two 25 mm long tibial tunnels are drilled, according to the size of the graft. The graft is then pulled into the femoral tunnel and fixed with an interference screw. The free ends of the allograft are then passed down the soft tissue plane and retrieved from the tibial incision. The posterior bundle is fixed with an interference screw with the knee in internal rotation and 60° of flexion (Fig. 6.7). The anterior bundle is fixed in the same way but with the knee flexed at 30° [27].

6.7 Tips to Find the Isometric Point

Finding the isometric point on the tibia, but mostly on the femur, is essential in order to achieve good stability and avoid stiffness after MCL reconstruction. Four different methods can be used to find the isometric points:

1. Two K wires can be positioned at the presumptive isometric points. A suture is then looped around the K wires and held with a Kelly clamp. In case of isometricity the suture should have the same tension throughout full range of motion (Fig. 6.8).
2. Alternatively, when the hamstring autograft is left attached distally, a K wire is positioned at the isometric point on the femur; the graft is looped around it and marked with a surgical marker. The knee is then taken through a full range of motion (Fig. 6.9). Displacement of the marks with respect to the K wire greater than 2 mm indicates a non-isometric point on the femur [22].
3. The graft can be looped around the K wire positioned at the presumptive isometric point on the femur and held with a Kelly clamp. If the graft is isometric, uniform tension throughout full range of motion can be appreciated with a probe (Fig. 6.10).
4. Fluoroscopy is used to obtain a perfect lateral view of the distal femur. The isometric point is located where the Blumensaat's line intersects the line of the anterior aspect of the posterior femoral shaft cortex [28, 29].

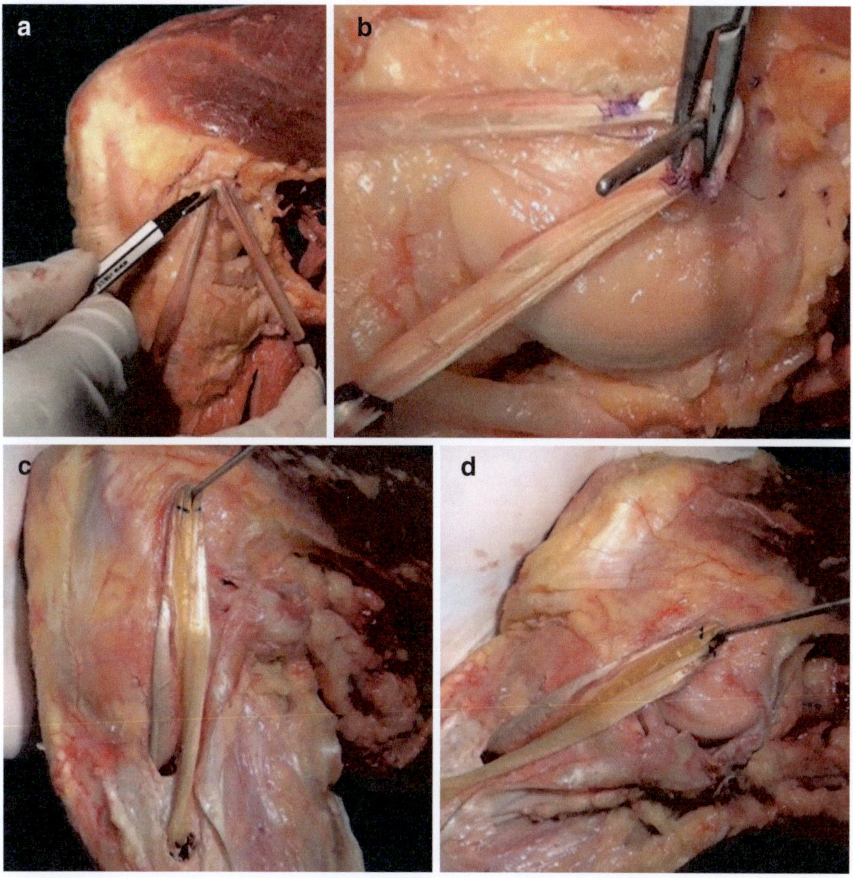

Fig. 6.9 Technique to find the isometric points. When the hamstring graft is left attached distally, a K wire is positioned at the isometric point on the femur; the graft is looped around it and marked with a surgical pen (**a**). The knee is then taken through a full range of motion. Displacement of the marks with respect to the K wire greater than 2 mm indicates a non isometric point on the femur (**b**). Note that the marks are not moving in case of isometricity, while the knee is brought from flexion (**c**) to extension (**d**)

6.8 Authors' Preferred Technique

Authors' preferred technique is Kim's procedure. This technique is easy (no need for multiple tunnel drilling), reliable (good results described in the literature), inexpensive (only one fixation device), and reproducible and allows for both sMCL and POL reconstruction.

6.9 Postoperative Management

Although standard rehabilitation protocols are not available, the authors' postoperative regimen is as follows. The patient is kept in a hinged knee brace with partial weight bearing. Passive range of motion from 0° to 90° is begun immediately.

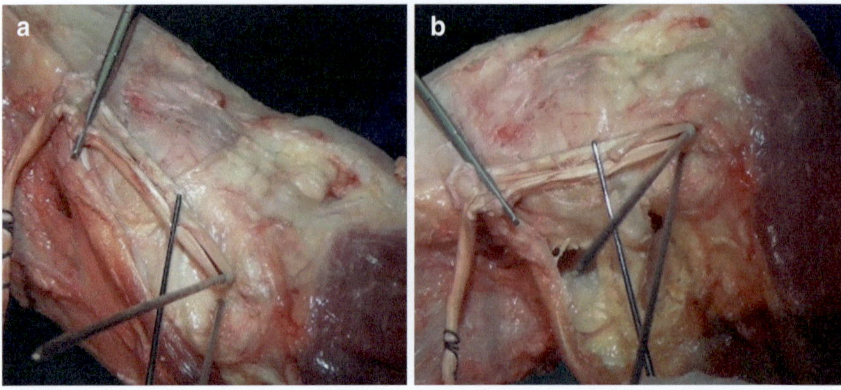

Fig. 6.10 Technique to find the isometric points. The graft can be looped around the K wire positioned at the presumptive isometric point on the femur and held with a Kelly clamp. If the graft is isometric, uniform tension throughout a full range of motion can be appreciated with a probe (**a**, **b**)

Hyperextension and flexion over 90° should be avoided during the first 2 weeks. Isometric strengthening is allowed immediately. Full range of motion is allowed 3 weeks after surgery together with closed kinetic chain strengthening; full weight bearing is allowed 6 weeks after surgery. Return to full activities is generally at 4–6 months after surgery.

6.10 Results

Good results have been reported in the acute and chronic setting after PMC reconstruction procedures [22, 24, 29].

A review of the recent studies describing the outcomes of MCL and PMC reconstruction is summarized in Table 6.1. Rare postoperative complications were reported for each technique. Out of 24 patients, Kim described 1 case of wound infection and 2 cases of late loosening of a screw. Lind described 1case of septic arthritis and slight knee ROM reduction in overall 20 % of the patients.

However, the limitations of the literature regarding this topic are evident. As shown in the outcome table, the studies available are mostly case series, with heterogeneous study groups (with or without associated ligamentous injuries), and different medial laxity grading systems or outcome scores.

6.11 Discussions and Conclusions

MCL and PMC injuries are relatively common [30]. PMC injuries are common in high-energy traumas (i.e., multiligament knee), whereas isolated MCL injury is usually combined with ACL tears. Understanding of the anatomy of the medial side of the knee, correct indications, and precise surgical techniques are essential in

Table 6.1 Outcomes of MCL/PMC reconstruction

Author, year, and reference	Number of patients and type of injury	Technique	Graft used	Follow-up	Outcomes
Kim et al. (2008) [22]	24 MCL + POL	Reconstruction MCL/PMC	Semitendinosus autograft with preserved tibial attachment	Mean 52.6 months (range 25–92)	Lysholm score 91.9 (range 80–100) 2 mm medial joint space opening in 22/24
Lind et al. (2009) [24]	13 isolated MCL 34 ACL + MCL 14 multiple ligaments	Reconstruction MCL/PMC	Semitendinosus autograft with preserved tibial attachment	Median 40 months (range 26–68)	91.2 % of subjective satisfaction 98 % of normal or nearly normal knee stability
Stannard et al. (2012) [29]	73 patients with knee dislocation	25 repairs vs 48 reconstructions of MCL and POL	Semitendinosus autograft or allograft reconstruction	Mean 43 months	5 failures (20 %) in the repair group 2 failures (4 %) in the reconstruction group

MCL medial collateral ligament, *PMC* posteromedial corner, *ACL* anterior cruciate ligament, *PCL* posterior cruciate ligament order to achieve good results. Many surgical techniques have been described for MCL/PMC reconstruction. However, the literature is sparse regarding this topic and no technique has shown superior results over the others. When performing a MCL/PMC reconstruction, evaluation of limb alignment and combined ligamentous injuries is essential in order to plan a successful surgery. In case of valgus alignment and chronic medial instability, distal femoral varus osteotomy should be considered. Intraoperatively, we emphasize the importance of finding the isometric point (mostly on the femur) in order to avoid knee stiffness, which can be probably considered the most common complication in this type of surgery.

References

1. Pedowitz RA, O'Connor JJ, Akeson WH (2003) Daniel's knee injuries: ligament and cartilage structure, function, injury, and repair, 2nd edn. Lippincott Williams & Wilkins, Philadelphia
2. Tibor LM, Marchant MH Jr, Taylor DC, Hardaker WT Jr, Garrett WE Jr, Sekiya JK (2011) Management of medial-sided knee injuries, part 2: posteromedial corner. Am J Sports Med 39–6:1332–1340
3. Mueller W (1983) The knee: form, function, and ligament reconstruction. Springer, Berlin
4. Robinson JR, Sanchez-Ballester J, Bull AM, Thomas Rde W, Amis AA (2004) The posteromedial corner revisited: an anatomical description of the passive restraining structures of the medial aspect of the human knee. J Bone Joint Surg Br 86–B:674–681
5. Haimes JL, Wroble RR, Grood ES et al (1994) Role of the medial structures in the intact and anterior cruciate ligament-deficient knee. Limits of motion in the human knee. Am J Sports Med 22:402–409
6. Griffith CJ, LaPrade RF, Johansen S, Armitage BM, Wijdicks CA, Engebresten L (2009) Medial knee injury: part 1, static function of the individual components of the main medial knee structures. Am J Sports Med 37:1762–1770
7. Petersen W, Loerch S, Schanz S et al (2008) The role of the posterior oblique ligament in controlling posterior tibial translation in the posterior cruciate ligament deficient knee. Am J Sports Med 36:495–501
8. Fetto JF, Marshall JL (1978) Medial collateral ligament injuries of the knee: a rationale for treatment. Clin Orthop 132:206–218
9. Fanelli GC, Harris JD (2006) Surgical treatment of acute medial collateral ligament and posteromedial corner injuries of the knee. Sports Med Arthrosc 14(2):78–83
10. Robinson JR, Bull AMJ, Thomas RR, Amis AA (2006) The role of the medial collateral ligament and posteromedial capsule in controlling knee laxity. Am J Sports Med 34:1815–1823
11. Bauer KL, Stannard JP (2013) Surgical approach to the posteromedial corner: indications, technique, outcomes. Curr Rev Musculoskelet Med 6(2):124–131
12. Lonner JH, Dupuy DE, Siliski JM (2000) Comparison of magnetic resonance imaging with operative findings in acute traumatic dislocations of the adult knee. J Orthop Trauma 14:183–186
13. Holden DL, Eggert AW, Butler JE (1983) The nonoperative treatment of grades I and II medial collateral ligament injuries to the knee. Am J Sports Med 11:340–344. 36
14. Indelicato PA, Hermansdorfer J, Huegel M (1990) Nonoperative management of complete tears of the medial collateral ligament of the knee in intercollegiate football players. Clin Orthop Relat Res 256:174–177
15. Klimkiewicz JJ, Petrie RS, Harner CD (2000) Surgical treatment of combined injury to anterior cruciate ligament, posterior cruciate ligament and medial structures. Clin Sports Med 19:479–492

16. Levy BA, Fanelli GC, Whelan DB, Stannard JP, MacDonald PA, Boyd JL, et al, Knee Dislocation Study Group (2009) Controversies in the treatment of knee dislocation and multiligament reconstruction. J Am Acad Orthop Surg 17(4):197–206
17. Bonasia DE, Bruzzone M, Dettoni F, Marmotti A, Blonna D, Castoldi F, Gasparetto F, D'Elicio D, Collo G, Rossi R (2012) Treatment of medial and posteromedial knee instability: indications, techniques, and review of the results. Iowa Orthop J 32:173–183. Review
18. Noyes FR, Barber-Westin SD (2005) Posterior cruciate ligament revision reconstruction, part 1: causes of failure in 52 consecutive operations. Am J Sports Med 33:646–654
19. Peterson W, Loerch S, Schanz S, Raschke M, Zantop T (2008) The role of the posterior oblique ligament in controlling posterior tibial translation in the posterior cruciate ligament-deficient knee. Am J Sports Med 36:493–501
20. Benjamin JJ 3rd, Ferguson CM, Martin DF (2006) Surgical treatment of chronic posteromedial instability using capsular procedures. Sports Med Arthrosc 14(2):91–95
21. Hughston JC, Barrett GR (1983) Acute anteromedial rotatory instability. Long-term results of surgical repair. J Bone Joint Surg Am 65(2):145–153
22. Kim SJ, Lee DH, Kim TE, Choi NH (2008) Concomitant reconstruction of the medial collateral and posterior oblique ligaments for medial instability of the knee. J Bone Joint Surg Br 90(10):1323–1327
23. Stannard JP (2010) Medial and posteromedial instability of the knee: evaluation, treatment, and results. Sports Med Arthrosc 18(4):263–268
24. Lind M, Jakobsen BW, Lund B, Hansen MS, Abdallah O, Christiansen SE (2009) Anatomical reconstruction of the medial collateral ligament and posteromedial corner of the knee in patients with chronic medial collateral ligament instability. Am J Sports Med 37(6):1116–1122
25. Coobs BR, Wijdicks CA, Armitage BM, Spiridonov SI, Westerhaus BD, Johansen S, Engebretsen L, Laprade RF (2010) An in vitro analysis of an anatomical medial knee reconstruction. Am J Sports Med 38:339–347
26. Wijdicks CA, Griffith CJ, Johansen S, Engebretsen L, Laprade RF (2010) Injuries to the medial collateral ligament and associated medial structures of the knee. J Bone Joint Surg Am 92(5):1266–1280
27. Borden PS, Kantaras AT, Caborn DN (2002) Medial collateral ligament reconstruction with allograft using a double-bundle technique. Arthroscopy 18(4):E19
28. Stannard JP, Bauer KL (2012) Current concepts in knee dislocations: PCL, ACL, and medial sided injuries. J Knee Surg 25:287–294
29. Stannard JS, Black BS, Azbell C, Volgas DA (2012) Posteromedial corner injury in knee dislocations. J Knee Surg 25:429–434
30. Sims WF, Jacobsen KE (2004) The posteromedial corner of the knee: medial-sided injury patterns revisited. Am J Sports Med 32:337–345

Chronic Anterolateral Knee Laxity: Reconstruction Techniques

7

Patrick Djian, Romain Rousseau, and Konstantinos G. Makridis

7.1 Introduction

Lateral extra-articular reconstructions were used as isolated procedures in knees with moderate rotatory instability. Nowadays, lateral reconstructions are used as additional procedures in knees requiring primary repair or intra-articular reconstruction for major rotatory instability.

Normal knee joint kinematics, particularly rotational stability, are not fully restored performing a single-bundle anterior cruciate ligament (ACL) reconstruction [21, 45]. A failure rate ranging from 11 to 30 % has been reported in the literature [5, 23, 28]. Different techniques have been proposed to improve ACL reconstruction [4, 17, 32, 48]. Anatomic double-bundle reconstruction, reproducing the anteromedial (AM) and posterolateral (PL) bundles, has been introduced to better control knee rotation [39, 47]. Extra-articular procedures such as lateral tenodesis have been proposed to reduce the rotational laxity [8].

These extra-articular procedures aim to prevent pivot shift and protect the intra-articular graft by a load-sharing mechanism, while the graft tissue is remodeling.

Sydney et al. [44] in a cadaveric knee experiment have shown that an iliotibial band tenodesis reduces the occurrence of the pivot shift phenomenon and decreases the displacement in Lachman test by holding the tibia in a position of external rotation during flexion. They have demonstrated that tenodesis was nonfunctional at extension, taut between 20° and 60°, and overly tight at 90° of flexion, which may potentially be the reason why tenodesis sometimes stretches out and becomes clinically ineffective over time.

In 1990, L. Engebretsen et al. [16] showed in another cadaveric study that the combination of an iliotibial band tenodesis with a standard intra-articular reconstruction significantly decreased the force in the ACL composite graft by an average of 43 %.

P. Djian (✉) • R. Rousseau • K.G. Makridis
Department of Orthopedic, Clinic Cabinet Goethe, 23 Avenue Niel, Paris 75017, France
e-mail: patrick.djian@wanadoo.fr

R. Rossi, F. Margheritini (eds.), *Knee Ligament Injuries*,
DOI 10.1007/978-88-470-5513-1_7, © Springer Verlag Italia 2014

In 1993, Amis and Scammell [4] reported in their cadaveric study that there is no significant biomechanical advantage from adding an extra-articular reconstruction in an isolated ACL-deficient knee.

In 1996, Samuelson et al. [41] performed another cadaveric study. When a tenodesis with either 0 N or 22 N of tension was added to the intra-articular reconstruction in knees with combined injuries, the excessive internal rotation significantly decreased at all angles of flexion, but not at full extension with 0 N of tension. Authors recommended to use tenodesis when the laxity is important or combined with rotational instability.

The purpose of this chapter is to describe the different reconstruction techniques used in anterolateral knee laxity and review their efficacy and results in the literature.

7.2 Surgical Techniques

Several different techniques for extra-articular reconstruction have been described. Most of them use strips of isolated iliotibial band (ITB) to act as a restraint to internal rotation of the tibia and to anterior laxity of the lateral compartment.

Lemaire Procedure (Fig. 7.1). This technique was first described in 1967 [29]. A 15 cm × 1.5 cm strip of fascia lata attached to Gerdy's tubercle was passed under the lateral collateral ligament and then through a bone tunnel at the lateral head of gastrocnemius. It was then passed again under the lateral collateral ligament before being attached through another bony tunnel under Gerdy's tubercle [28, 36].

Christel and Djian [7] (Fig. 7.2) have described a short strip of iliotibial band with a bone tunnel in the femur. Tenodesis consists of a 12 × 75 mm strip of ITB remaining attached to Gerdy's tubercle. An isometric point in the region of Krackow's point F9 [26] is determined with a caliper. The strip is twisted by 180° to enhance isometry. Then it is fixed through a tunnel drilled in the femur. The fixation is achieved by an interference screw.

MacIntosh Procedure (Fig. 7.3). This procedure [24] used a strip of ITB in a technique called the lateral substitution reconstruction. A 20 cm long strip, 2–4 cm in width, was dissected from the mid-portion of the ITB and turned down to its attachment at Gerdy's tubercle. A subperiosteal tunnel was made in the lateral femoral

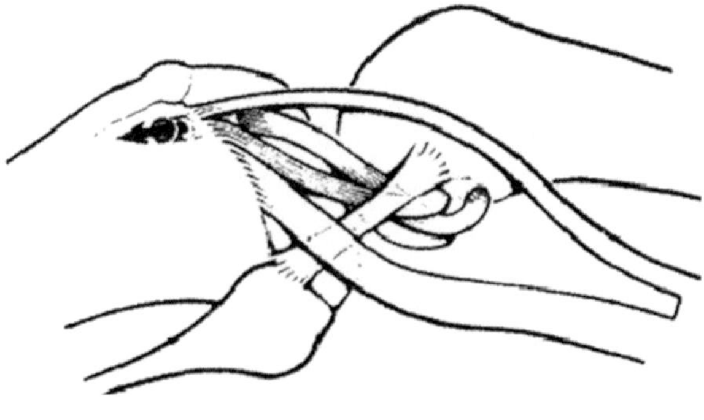

Fig. 7.1 Lemaire procedure [29]. Lateral extra articular reconstruction with a strip of ITB passed through the lateral condyle and under le lateral collateral ligament

condyle posterior to the attachment of the fibular collateral ligament. The strip of ITB was passed deep to the collateral ligament and through the periosteal tunnel. A second subperiosteal tunnel was made to insert the strip of ITB through the distal insertion of the lateral intermuscular septum onto the lateral femoral condyle. The band was looped behind the insertion of the intermuscular septum and then passed again deep to the collateral ligament. The ITB was then anchored with the knee held at 90° flexion.

Losee's Procedure (Fig. 7.4). Losee et al. [31] designed an operation again using a strip of ITB. An incision was made approximately 15 cm proximal to the knee joint. Then, several parallel incisions, 2.5 cm apart, were performed in the ITB to obtain a strip of tissue approximately 16 cm long, which was remained attached to Gerdy's tubercle. A tunnel was made through the lateral femoral condyle, anterior and distal to the attachment of the lateral collateral ligament, followed by passage of the ITB graft.

Ellison's Distal ITB Transfer (Fig. 7.5). Ellison's technique [15] was a modification of earlier work by Galway and MacIntosh [20], but the ITB was released from its origin at Gerdy's tubercle, before being passed under the insertion of the lateral collateral ligament to the femoral condyle.

Andrews's Operation (Fig. 7.6). This procedure was a mini reconstruction designed to prevent anterolateral instability, using isometric bundles in the ITB [1, 2]. Two extra-articular strips of ITB were fixed to the lateral condyle so that the anterior strip was tight in flexion and the posterior tight in extension.

Müller ALFTL Tenodesis [35]. This tenodesis was performed by surgically isolating a 1.25 cm strip from the posterior portion of the iliotibial tract. The strip was

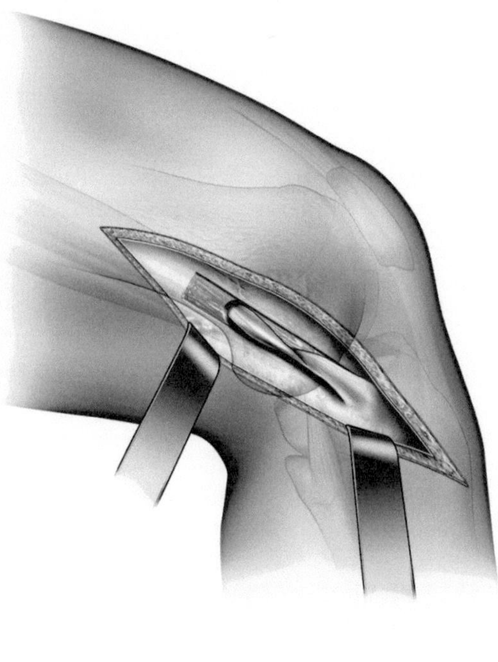

Fig. 7.2 Extra articular tenodesis [7]. Lateral extra articular reconstruction with a strip of ITB passed through the condyle

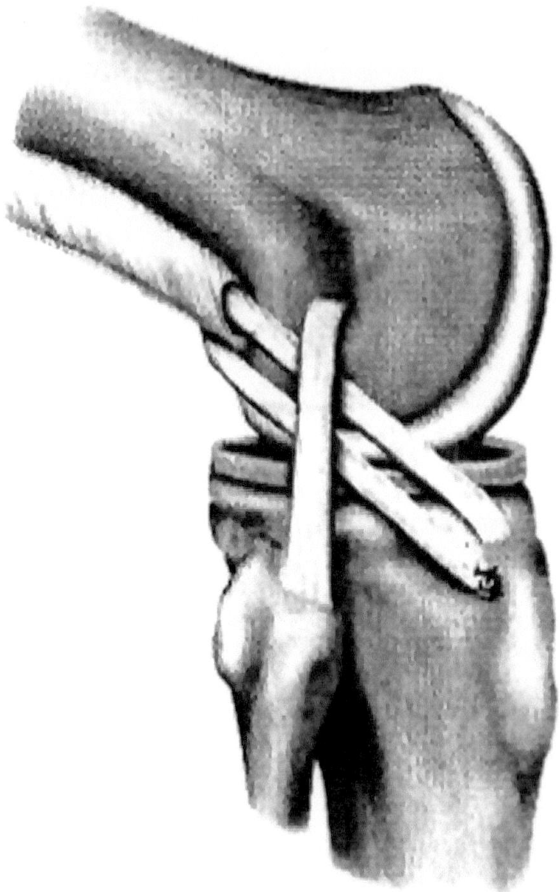

Fig. 7.3 MacIntosh procedure [24]. Lateral extra articular reconstruction with a strip of ITB passed through the intermuscular septum and under le lateral collateral ligament

created with two parallel fiber-splitting incisions, preserving its distal attachment to the rest of the iliotibial tract. A clinically isometric point of attachment for this strip was selected at the junction of the femoral shaft and lateral femoral condyle in the locus corresponding to Krackow's point F9 [26]. This point is somewhat distal and posterior to that illustrated in Müller monograph 2′ and was chosen in order to easier achieve a clinical isometry at this anatomical site. The strip was then fixed using a 3.5 mm AO fully threaded cancellous screw and a toothed washer.

Combined Intra- and Extra-articular Reconstruction. Extra-articular techniques have been used to augment an intra-articular reconstruction, because it was supposed to protect the intra-articular graft during the healing phase.

Marcacci's [32] technique included hamstrings graft as an intra-articular reconstruction combined with an extra-articular augmentation (Fig. 7.5). Semitendinosus and gracilis tendons were harvested but left attached to the tibia. They were passed through the tibial and femoral tunnels, before being passed laterally and then deep

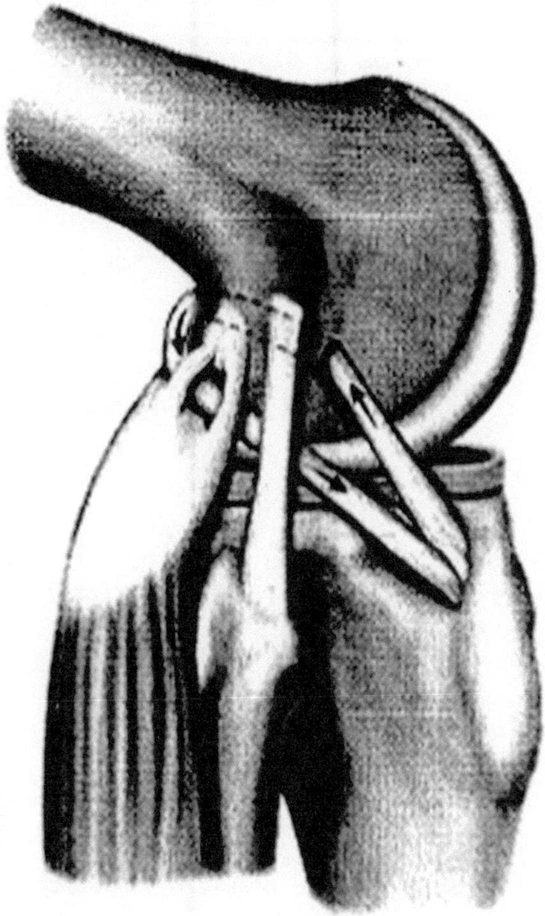

Fig. 7.4 Losee procedure [31]. The graft is passed through an extra articular tunnel on the femur and through the capsule and the lateral gastrocnemius

to the ITB to be fixed onto Gerdy's tubercle. With this technique, problems associated with ITB graft, such as donor site morbidity, were avoided.

Other authors have described similar techniques using extra-articular tenodesis with the same hamstring grafts [6, 8].

Roth et al. [40] compared isolated intra-articular with combined intra- and extra-articular reconstruction. They concluded that there was no benefit in using an additional extra-articular repair. However, there were no clear indications why some patients were selected to have an isolated intra- articular reconstruction and some others a combined procedure.

Strum et al. [43] compared 43 patients who had a combined repair with 84 who had an isolated intra-articular reconstruction. No difference was found in treatment outcome. Similarly, other studies have shown no benefit of an additional extra-articular reconstruction [4, 37].

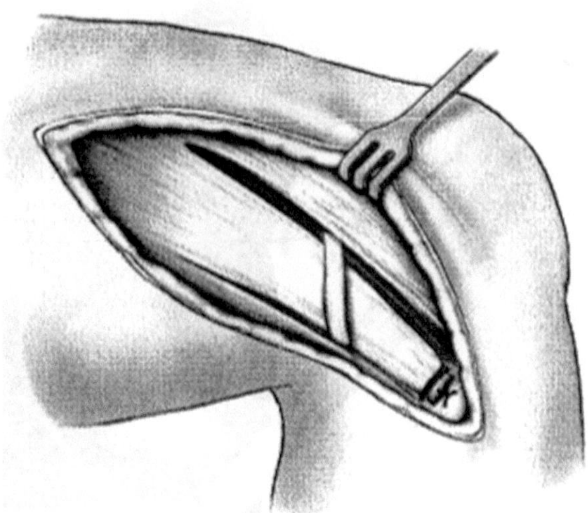

Fig. 7.5 Ellison procedure [15]. The ilio tibial band is passed under the lateral collateral ligament. The ITB is intact proximally

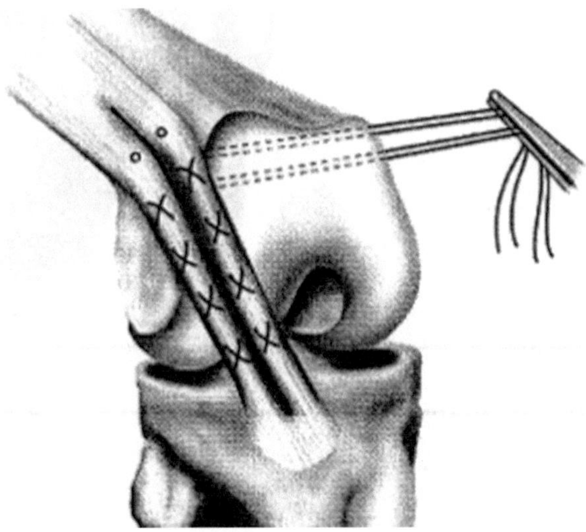

Fig. 7.6 Andrew procedure [1, 2]. Two extra articular strips of ITB are fixed to the lateral condyle so the anterior strip is tight in flexion and the posterior strip is tight in extension

7.3 Results

Results are shown in Table 7.1.

7.4 Discussion

Lateral extra-articular reconstruction has been undertaken either as an isolated procedure or to augment an intra-articular reconstruction.

Table 7.1 Results of isolated extra-articular anterior cruciate ligament reconstruction

Authors	Technique	N of patients	Follow-up	Postop protocol	Scoring system	Outcome
Amirault et al. [3]	MacIntosh technique	27	11.3 years (8–14)	Long leg cast 5 weeks	Clinical assessment	52 % excellent or good 26 % fair 22 % poor
Dandy [9]	MacIntosh technique	18	69 months		Lysholm	
Durkan et al. [11]	Ellison procedure	104	51 months (24–100)	Long leg cast 6 weeks	Subjective and clinical assessment	80 % excellent and good 14 % fair results 6 % poor results
Ellison [15]	ITB	18		Long leg cast 6 weeks	Kennedy	44 % excellent 39 % good 17 % failures
Frank and Jackson [18]	MacIntosh technique	35	12 years	Long leg cast 6 weeks	Clinical assessment	77 % excellent 17 % slightly better 6 % poor results
Fox et al. [19]	Ellison procedure	76				
Hanks et al. [22]	Ellison procedure	30	25 months	Long leg cast 6 weeks	Objective and subjective assessment	79 % good subjectively 46 % good objectively
Ireland and Trickey [24]	MacIntosh technique	50	2.2 years	Long leg cast 6 weeks	Clinical assessment	
Kennedy et al. [25]	Ellison procedure	28	6 months	Long leg cast 6 weeks	Subjective assessment	57 % excellent or good results 24 had pivot shift
Lazzarone et al. [27]	Lemaire procedure	40				80 % excellent and good results
Losee et al. [31]	Losee procedure	50	1–6.5 years	Long leg cast 7 weeks	Subjective and objective assessment	41 good 6 fair 3 poor

(continued)

Table 7.1 (continued)

Authors	Technique	N of patients	Follow-up	Postop protocol	Scoring system	Outcome
Marston and Chen [33]	Ellison technique	22	59 months	Long leg cast 6 weeks	Clinical assessment	77 % excellent
Molster et al. [34]	Losee technique	34	2 (1–4)	Long leg cast 6 weeks	Lysholm	61 % excellent and good results
Neyret et al. [36]	Lemaire	33	4.5 years		Arpege score subjective and clinical assessment	
Taylor et al. [46]	MacIntosh	18	Mean 9.3 months	Long leg cast 4 weeks	Cincinnati	
Reid et al. [38]	Ellison	32	11 years (7–15)		Lysholm	

Some authors have reported failure of the extra-articular reconstruction and recurrent instability [3, 9, 31, 43]. Degenerative changes caused by lateral compartment overtightening have been reported [37, 43]. However, these procedures were performed without concomitant intra-articular ACL reconstruction, probably allowing the joint to be secured in a subluxed posterolateral position. Another possible cause for the poor postoperative function might be the rehabilitation methods employed, which included long-standing postoperative immobilization of the knee [9, 42].

7.4.1 Tips and Tricks to Avoid Problems Using Lateral Extra-articular Reconstruction Techniques

The exact site of femoral attachment and tension of the extra-articular reconstruction is critical in determining the successful restoration of normal biomechanics. It has been suggested that the optimum site of femoral fixation is proximal and posterior to the femoral origin of the lateral collateral ligament. The lack of reproducibility could be due to variability in determining the fixation site of the tenodesis on the femoral condyle among the specimens, although the authors aimed for Krackow's F9 site posterior and proximal to the insertion of the lateral collateral ligament [30]. The use of caliper during the procedure facilitates the Krackow's F9 exact site.

A 180° twist modeled into the tenodesis significantly reduced the range of changes in distance (difference between the largest and smallest changes in distance among the lines for a given angle of flexion) for both of these load states [12, 13]. Therefore, a 180° twist in the tenodesis can enhance isometry among the fibers of the tenodesis. This implies that a 180° twist can enhance load sharing among the fibers of the tenodesis and, therefore, enhance the overall strength of the tenodesis.

The ITB screw tenodesis was ineffective in reducing anterior translation of the tibia in the anterior cruciate ligament-deficient knee at forces approximating in vivo conditions [4, 16]. Significant stretching and tearing of the tract occurred around the screw under these testing conditions, a finding that helps explain the possible initial success and later failure of an isolated extra-articular procedure. The fixation by washer and screw is not recommended. We [7] developed a technique with a bone tunnel and a fixation by a screw [14]. This technique is reproducible.

Finally, positioning of the knee in terms of flexion and external rotation is also critical. The fixation must be done at 30° of flexion and without any external rotation of the tibia [12, 13].

Conclusion

Intra-articular ACL reconstruction is an effective procedure [10]. Attempts to improve its results and obtain a better restoration of kinematics should address the extra-articular structures that contribute to the pivot shift phenomenon. However, further improvements of these extra-articular techniques are necessary to provide better biomechanical fixation and reduce failure and revision rates when used in conjunction with intra-articular reconstruction.

Overtightening and fixation in a posterolateral drawer position is not recommended, because this position can lead to degenerative changes in the lateral knee compartment.

A prolonged knee immobilization is not recommended and an immediate rehabilitation schedule is strongly advised.

References

1. Andrews JR, Sanders RA, Morin B (1985) Surgical treatment of anterolateral instability: a follow-up study. Am J Sports Med 13:112–119
2. Andrews JR, Sanders R (1983) A "mini-reconstruction" technique in treating anterolateral rotatory instability (ALRI). Clin Orthop 172:93–96
3. Amirault JD, Cameron JC, MacIntosh DL, Marks P (1988) Chronic anterior cruciate ligament deficiency: long-term results of MacIntosh's lateral substitution reconstruction. J Bone Joint Surg [Br] 70-B:622–624
4. Amis AA, Scammell BE (1993) Biomechanics of intra-articular and extra- articular reconstruction of the anterior cruciate ligament. J Bone Joint Surg Br 75(5):812–817
5. Bach BR Jr, Tradonsky S, Bojchuk J, Levy ME, Bush-Joseph CA, Khan NH (1998) Arthroscopically assisted anterior cruciate ligament reconstruction using patellar tendon autograft: five- to nine-year follow-up evaluation. Am J Sports Med 26(1):20–29
6. Burgot D, Rosset P, Favard L, Burdin P (1988) Chronic anterior laxity of the knee treated by extra-articular ligamentoplasty: 226 cases reviewed after more than 2 years. Rev Chir Orthop Reparatrice Appar Mot 74:424–429
7. Christel P, Djian P (2002) Anterio-lateral extra-articular tenodesis of the knee using a short strip of fascia lata. Rev Chir Orthop Reparatrice Appar Mot 88(5):508–513
8. Colombet P (2011) Knee laxity control in revision anterior cruciate ligament reconstruction versus anterior cruciate ligament reconstruction and lateral tenodesis: clinical assessment using computer-assisted navigation. Am J Sports Med 39:1248
9. Dandy DJ (1995) Some clinical aspects of reconstruction for chronic anterior cruciate ligament deficiency. Ann R Coll Surg Engl 77:290–298
10. Dodds AL, Gupte CM, Neyret P, Williams AM, Amis AA (2011) Extra-articular techniques in anterior cruciate ligament reconstruction. A literature review. J Bone Joint Surg Br 93-B:1440–1448
11. Durkan JA, Wynne GF, Haggerty JF (1989) Extraarticular reconstruction of the anterior cruciate ligament insufficient knee. A long-term analysis of the Ellison procedure. Am J Sports Med 17(1):112–117
12. Draganich LF, Reider B, Miller PR (1989) An in vitro study of the Muller antero-lateral femorotibial ligament tenodesis in the anterior cruciate ligament deficient knee. Am J Sports Med 17:357–362
13. Draganich LF, Reider B, Ling M et al (1990) An in vitro of an intraarticular Draganich Ling study and extraarticular reconstruction in the anterior cruciate ligament deficient knee. Am J Sports Med 18:262–266
14. Draganich LF, Hsieh YE, Reider B (1995) Iliotibial band tenodesis: a new strategy for attachment. Am J Sports Med 23(2):186–195
15. Ellison AE (1979) Distal iliotibial-band transfer for anterolateral rotator instability of the knee. J Bone Joint Surg Am 61-A:330–337
16. Engebretsen L, Lew WD, Lewis JL, Hunter RE (1990) The effect of an iliotibial tenodesis on intraarticular graft forces and knee joint motion. Am J Sports Med 18(2):169–176
17. Ferretti A, Conteduca F, Monaco E, De Carli A, D'Arrigo C (2006) Revision anterior cruciate ligament reconstruction with doubled semitendinosus and gracilis tendons and lateral extra-articular reconstruction. J Bone Joint Surg Am 88(11):2373–2379

18. Frank C, Jackson RW (1988) Lateral substitution for chronic isolated anterior cruciate ligament deficiency. J Bone Joint Surg Br 70 B(3):407–411
19. Fox JM, Blazina ME, Del Pizzo W, Ivey FM, Broukhim B (1980) Extra articular stabilization of the knee joint for anterior instability. Clin Orthop Relat Res 147:56–61
20. Galway RD, Beaupre A, MacIntosh DL (1972) Pivot shift: a clinical sign of symptomatic anterior cruciate insufficiency. J Bone Joint Surg [Br] 54-B:763–764
21. Georgoulis AD, Papadonikolakis A, Papageorgiou CD, Mitsou A, Stergiou N (2003) Three-dimensional tibiofemoral kinematics of the anterior cruciate ligament-deficient and reconstructed knee during walking. Am J Sports Med 31(1):75–79
22. Hanks GA, Joyner DM, Kalenak A (1981) Antero lateral rotatory instability of the knee. An analysis of the Ellison procedure. Am J Sports Med 9(4):225–232
23. Harter RA, Osternig LR, Singer KM, James SL, Larson RL, Jones DC (1988) Long-term evaluation of knee stability and function following surgical reconstruction for anterior cruciate ligament insufficiency. Am J Sports Med 16(5):434–443
24. Ireland J, Trickey EL (1980) Macintosh tenodesis for anterolateral instability of the knee. J Bone Joint Surg [Br] 62-B:340–345
25. Kennedy JC, Stewart R, Walker DM (1978) Anterolateral rotatory instability of the knee joint. J Bone Joint Surg Am 60-A:1031–1039
26. Krackow KA, Brooks RL (1983) Optimization of knee ligament position for lateral extraarticular reconstruction. Am J Sports Med 11:293–302
27. Lazzarone C, Crova M, Brach Del Prever E, Comba D (1990) Extraarticular reconstruction in the treatment of chronic lesions of the anterior cruciate ligament. Ital J Orthop Traumatol 16:459–465
28. Lebel B, Hulet C, Galaud B, Burdin G, Locker B, Vielpeau C (2008) Arthro- scopic reconstruction of the anterior cruciate ligament using bone- patellar tendon-bone autograft: a minimum 10-year follow-up. Am J Sports Med 36(7):1275–1282
29. Lemaire M (1967) Ruptures anciennes du ligament croise anterieur du genou. J Chir 93:311–320
30. Lipscombs AB, Woods W, Jones A (1992) A biomechanical evaluation of the iliotibial tract screw tenodesis. Am J Sports Med 20(6):742–745
31. Losee RE, Johnson TR, Southwick W (1978) Anterior subluxation of the lateral tibial plateau: a diagnostic test and operative repair. J Bone Joint Surg [Am] 60- A:1015–1030
32. Marcacci M, Zaffagnini S, Giordano G, Iacono F, Presti ML (2009) Anterior cruciate ligament reconstruction associated with extra-articular tenodesis: a prospective clinical and radiographic evaluation with 10- to 13-year follow-up. Am J Sports Med 37(4):707–714
33. Marston RA, Chen SC (1993) Extra articular tenodesis for anterior cruciate deficient knees: a review of Ellison procedure. J R Soc Med 86(11):637–638
34. Mølster AO, Strand T, Skredderstuen A, Engesaeter LB, Raugstad TS, Alho A (1984) Extra articular stabilization of the knee a.m Losee. Acta Orthop Scand 55(6):640–642
35. Muller W (1983) The knee: form, function, and ligament reconstruction. Springer, New York, pp 253–257
36. Neyret P, Palamo J, Donell ST, Dejour H (1994) Extra-articular tenodesis for anterior cruciate ligament rupture in amateur skiers. Br J Sports Med 28:31–34
37. O'Brien SJ, Warren RF, Pavlov H, Panariello R, Wickiewicz TL (1991) Reconstruction of the chronically insufficient anterior cruciate ligament with the central third of the patellar ligament. J Bone Joint Surg Am 73-A:278–286
38. Reid JS, Hanks GA, Kalanek A, Kottmeier S, Aronoff V (1992) The Ellison iliotibial- band transfer for a torn anterior cruciate ligament of the knee: long-term follow-up. J Bone Joint Surg Am 74-A:1392–1402
39. Robinson J, Carrat L, Granchi C, Colombet P (2007) Influence of anterior cruciate ligament bundles on knee kinematics: clinical assessment using computer-assisted navigation. Am J Sports Med 35(12):2006–2013
40. Roth JH, Kennedy JC, Lockstadt H, McCallum CL, Cunning LA (1987) Intra-articular reconstruction of the anterior cruciate ligament with and without extra-articular supplementation by transfer of the biceps femoris tendon. J Bone Joint Surg Am 69-A:275–278

41. Samuelson M, Draganich LF, Zhou X, Krumins P, Reider B (1996) The effects of knee reconstruction on combined anterior cruciate ligament and anterolateral capsular deficiencies. Am J Sports Med 24(4):492–497
42. Saragaglia D, Leroy JM, De Sousa B, Tourne Y, Abu al Zahab M (1995) Medium-term results of 173 ligamentoplasties of the anterior cruciate ligament using the MacIntosh technique reinforced by the Kennedy ligament augmentation device (LAD). Knee Surg Sports Traumatol Arthrosc 3:68–74
43. Strum G, Fox J, Ferkel R et al (1989) Intra-articular versus intra-articular and extra-articular reconstruction for chronic anterior cruciate ligament instability. Clin Orthop 245:188–198
44. Sydney SV, Haynes DW, Hungerford DS et al (1987) The altered kinematic effect of an iliotibial band tenodesis on the anterior cruciate deficient knee. Trans Orthop Res Soc 12:266
45. Tashman S, Collon D, Anderson K, Kolowich P, Anderst W (2004) Abnormal rotational knee motion during running after anterior cruciate ligament reconstruction. Am J Sports Med 32(4):975–983
46. Taylor GR, Fernandez GN, Robertson JA (1996) Long-term results of anterior cruciate reconstruction using a fascia lata graft. Knee 3:145–149
47. Yagi M, Wong EK, Kanamori A, Debski RE, Fu FH, Woo SL (2002) Biome- chanical analysis of an anatomic anterior cruciate ligament reconstruction. Am J Sports Med 30(5):660–666
48. Zaffagnini S, Marcacci M, Lo Presti M, Giordano G, Iacono F, Neri MP (2006) Prospective and randomized evaluation of ACL reconstruction with three techniques: a clinical and radiographic evaluation at 5 years follow-up. Knee Surg Sports Traumatol Arthrosc 14(11): 1060–1069

Chronic Lateral and Posterolateral Laxity: Reconstruction Techniques

8

Fabrizio Margheritini and Calogero Graci

8.1 Introduction

Chronic injury of the posterolateral corner (PLC) of the knee usually presents a more complex problem than acute injury because of extensive scarring, secondary changes to other structures, and possible limb malalignment. Thus, the treatment of these lesions represents a challenge for the surgeon.

Once an injury to the PLC has been detected, it is difficult to decide which treatment, conservative or surgical, is most appropriate. Historically isolated low-grade injuries to the posterolateral corner may do well with conservative treatment. On the opposite in more severe injuries, the outcome is poor [1]. The reason lies in the fact that chronic posterolateral injuries usually are the results of major trauma and frequently seen in combination with chronic cruciate ligament injuries. It has been shown either clinically or biomechanically that untreated grade 3 posterolateral corner injuries are a major cause of failure of cruciate ligament reconstructions. Therefore, it is recommended that grade 3 posterolateral corner injuries be repaired or reconstructed when anterior cruciate ligament or a posterior cruciate ligament reconstruction is done [2].

The indications for surgery include functional limitations, symptomatic instability and objective physical findings as a 2+ varus opening at 30° of knee flexion, a positivity to external rotation recurvatum test, posterolateral external rotation test, and dial test [3].

F. Margheritini (✉) • C. Graci
Department of Sports Sciences and Human Health,
Università degli studi di Roma "Foro Italico", IUSM,
Piazza Lauro de Bosis, 6, Rome 00135, Italy
e-mail: mararthro@gmail.com

R. Rossi, F. Margheritini (eds.), *Knee Ligament Injuries*,
DOI 10.1007/978-88-470-5513-1_8, © Springer Verlag Italia 2014

8.2 Surgical Techniques

Although a consensus exists on reconstructing the chronic posterolateral corner injury of the knee, there is a lack of consensus in the literature on the best technique of operative treatment [4].

Any reconstruction should focus on the most important posterolateral stabilizers: the lateral collateral ligament (LCL), the popliteus, and the peroneal-fibular ligament (PFL). Before proceeding with the reconstruction, the alignment of the knee should be assessed because varus malalignment can place excessive forces on any reconstruction if it is not corrected and a high tibial osteotomy (HTO) prior to soft tissue reconstruction may be required.

Sometimes the HTO itself, without others procedures, can resolve the symptoms of posterolateral instability [5].

There are numerous reconstruction options, including nonanatomic and anatomic ones.

Nonanatomic techniques for reconstructing the lateral side of the knee are now largely of historical importance since the advent of more anatomic reconstructive procedures.

Among nonanatomic chronic PLC techniques addressed to the popliteus insufficiency, surgical options include advancement and recession of its bony insertion, distal advancement, and tensioning of the tendon. Jakob et al. [6] recommended a recession of the popliteus tendon at its femoral insertion to restore mild posterolateral instability, but as with advancement of the arcuate complex, proximal recession will not restore adequate tension to the popliteus if there is distal injury at the musculotendinous junction or if there is injury of the popliteofibular ligament.

The surgical advancement is performed by removing the popliteus insertion with a bone plug and advancing and recessing it into a tunnel created at the original insertion site. The popliteus is then tensioned with the tibia in neutral rotation, and the sutures are tied over a button or bone bridge. The limit of this technique is that it can only be used when the popliteus tendon is still continuous and there is no evidence of injury at the musculotendinous junction in order to avoid failure caused by stretching. If injury occurred at the musculotendinous junction, but the popliteus tendon is strong, the preferred method is to tension the tendon by advancing it distally. This technique will remove the dynamic restraint because the tendon is fixed to the tibia.

Nonanatomic LCL reconstructions include, as the popliteus techniques, advancement and recession, biceps tendon augmentation, or substitution.

A recession may be performed by releasing the LCL from its femoral origin and either advancing it into a bone tunnel or securing it to its origin using a ligament washer. If a bone tunnel is used to reconstruct the popliteus tendon too, the LCL can be advanced into the posterior aspect of the same bone tunnel.

The biceps tendon may be used to augment the LCL if it is not injured. For augmentation of LCL with biceps tendon, the central two thirds of the biceps tendon is harvested by dissecting it from the muscle. The peroneal nerve is carefully identified and protected.

The strip of tendon is extended proximally and is left attached to the fibula distally. The isometric point on the femur is then located with suture and K-wire, and the harvested biceps tendon is turned up and secured to the femur using a ligament washer and screw.

Clancy [7] has used biceps tenodesis for reconstructing the posterolateral corner. The biceps tendon is transferred to the lateral femoral epicondyle, whereas its distal attachment to the fibula is left intact. The biceps tendon is freed from the lateral head of the gastrocnemius and the peroneal nerve. It is then passed under the split of the iliotibial band and attached with a ligament screw and washer to the lateral femoral epicondyle. This transfer recreates an LCL and may also tighten the arcuate complex. Because this reconstruction does not recreate the popliteus tendon or the popliteofibular ligament, it only represents a partial reconstruction of the injured structure.

Anatomic techniques, which attempt to restore the LCL, the PFL, and/or the popliteus, are subclassified into fibula-based and tibia-fibula-based procedures. Larson and coworkers proposed a fibula-based technique whereby a semitendinosus autograft is passed through an anterior-posterior drill hole in the fibula head, and both ends of the graft are then brought through a drilled socket in the lateral femoral epicondyle and fixed using an interference screw [8]. This method aims to reconstruct both the LCL and PFL. A modification of this technique, and our preferred technique, includes passing the two ends of the semitendinosus graft through two femoral sockets drilled at the attachment sites of the popliteus and LCL [9]. This allows restoration of the anatomic insertion of the popliteus, in addition to restoring the LCL and PFL.

Similarly, the goal of the tibia-fibula-based techniques is to restore all three anatomic structures. Veltri and Warren [10] also recommended that all injured posterolateral structures be anatomically reconstructed. A lateral collateral ligament with a chronic tear can usually be reconstructed with a section of biceps femoris tendon or, alternatively, with autograft or allograft. For tears that involve the popliteus complex, both the tibial and the fibular (popliteofibular ligament) attachments of the popliteus tendon should be addressed. With isolated injury of either the tibial or the fibular component of the popliteus complex, the surgeon can use a single graft fixed within the lateral femoral condyle that extends distally through a tunnel in the tibia or fibula, respectively. In cases where both the tibial and the fibular component of the popliteus complex are torn, a single split Achilles tendon allograft or patellar tendon autograft or allograft can be used [11].

Albright and Brown [12] described a posterolateral corner sling procedure for the treatment of posterolateral rotatory instability. Their technique involved use of an autograft, as a central slip of the iliotibial band, or an allograft to approximate reconstruction of the popliteus tendon and improve stability. The graft (acting as a sling) is passed through a tunnel in the proximal part of the tibia and is fixed just proximal to the origin of the lateral collateral ligament on the femoral condyle. Thirty patients had a combination of varus laxity and anterolateral or posterolateral rotatory instability prior to surgery. After 4 years of follow-up, eight patients (27 %) had an excellent result. Ten patients presented residual laxity, and six of these patients underwent additional stabilizing procedures that improved their outcome. The sling procedure was successful in eliminating the reverse pivot shift, hyperextension, and varus laxity in 26 of the 30 patients. This technique, however, does not include reconstruction of the lateral collateral ligament or the popliteofibular ligament [11].

Noyes and Barber-Westin [13] described a technique with the use of either a bone patellar tendon-bone autograft or allograft to reconstruct a deficient LCL in addition to reconstructing the popliteus arcuate complex with a semitendinosus and gracilis graft. They first reconstructed the LCL and performed either plication or advancement of the posterolateral structures, which were also sutured to the allograft LCL, producing a dense collagenous plate of tissues around the posterolateral corner of the knee.

LaPrade et al. more recently described a technique (specifically described elsewhere in this book), using two separate Achilles tendon-bone allografts through a fibula head tunnel, a lateral tibial plateau tunnel, and two femoral tunnels into which the bone blocks of the grafts are fixed [14].

While this new anatomic technique may be more appealing but more technically demanding than the fibula-based techniques, the best method for reconstruction of the LCL/PLC remains controversial from either a biomechanical or clinical viewpoint and thus without a clear gold standard.

8.3 Surgical Approach

A posterolateral reconstruction is usually done through a lateral approach to the knee. The author's preferred position is with the patient supine on the operative table with a lateral thigh post (Fig. 8.1). We believe that this position allows the best access and movement of the knee in a combined or isolated PLC reconstruction. The skin incision begins midway between the fibular head and Gerdy's tubercle (Fig. 8.2) and continues proximally to the lateral femoral epicondyle, paralleling the posterior edge of the iliotibial band for a total length of 12–15 cm. The peroneal nerve is identified proximally, posterior to the biceps tendon, and is dissected distally to the point at which it enters the anterior tibial muscular compartment (Fig. 8.3). If there is a peroneal palsy and hematoma is present within the nerve, the epineurium is released. Dissection is continued between the posterior edge of the iliotibial band and the biceps tendon, and the iliotibial band is split longitudinally allowing to retract posteriorly and anteriorly for further exposure. At this point, a vertical capsular incision can be made at the posterior border of the LCL allowing visualization of the lateral meniscus and popliteus tendon remnant, and all the PLC structures are evaluated systematically. At this point, a guide pin is next placed from anterior to posterior through the center of the fibular head at its area of maximum diameter (Fig. 8.4). A tunnel is next created through the fibular head, usually 5–6 mm in diameter. Drilling is usually directed toward a fingertip placed between the posterior aspect of the fibular head and the peroneal nerve. When the tunnel has been created, one end of the semitendinosus graft is passed through the tunnel, creating free ends exiting both the anterior and posterior aspects of the fibular head.

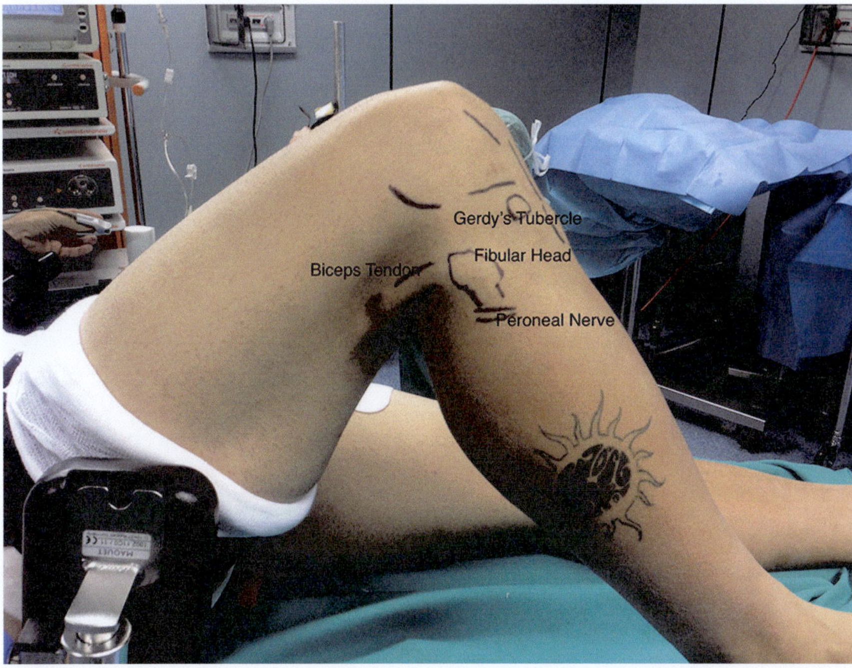

Fig. 8.1 Author's preferred position for isolated or combined PLC/cruciate ligaments reconstruction

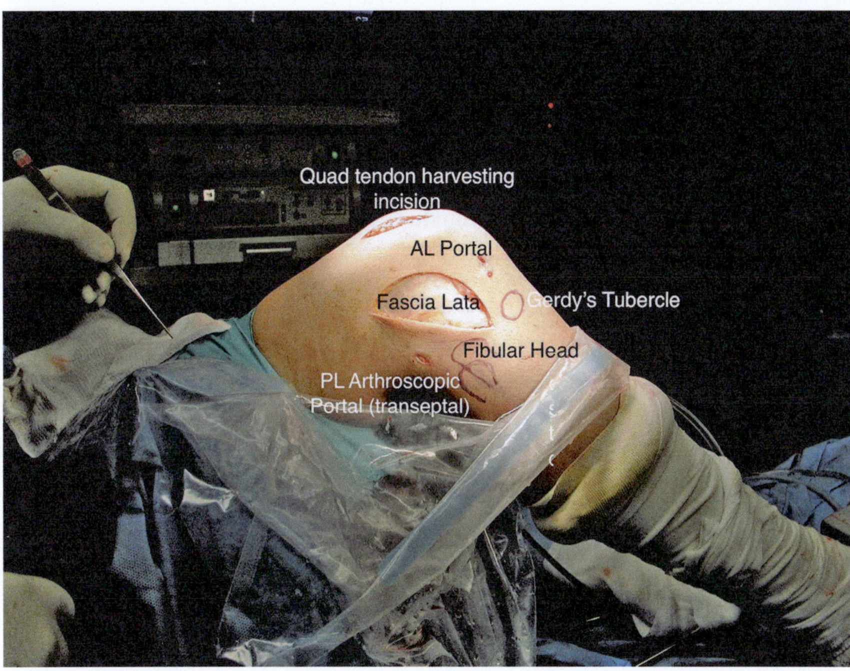

Fig. 8.2 Hockey's stick incision passing midway between Gerdy's tubercle and the peroneal head (Note: this patient had already harvested the quadriceps tendon for a PCL reconstruction)

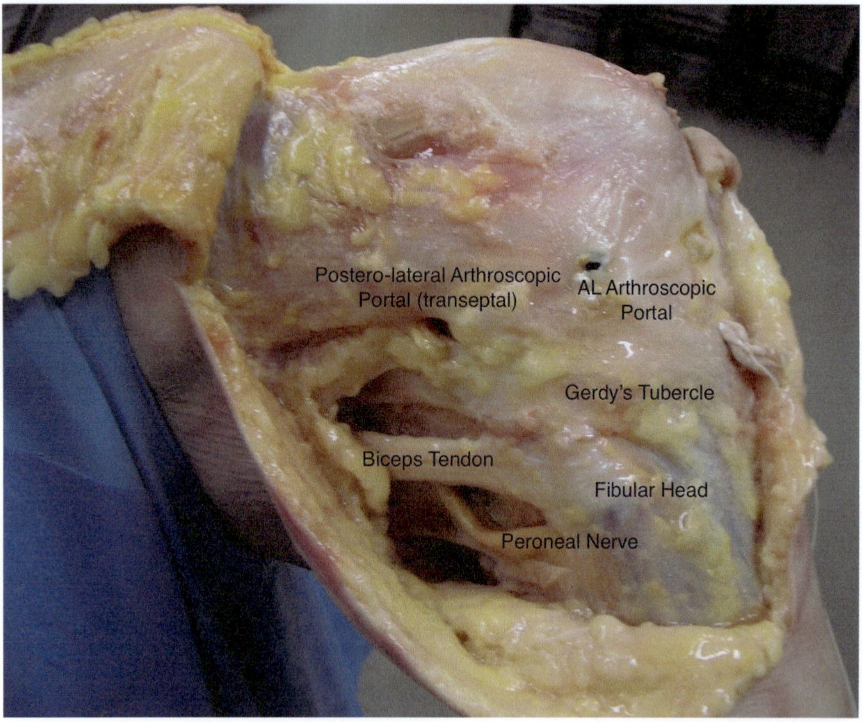

Fig. 8.3 Cadaveric specimen dissection showing the relations existing between the anatomical structures

Then an incision is made in the iliotibial band in line with its fibers directly overlying the lateral femoral epicondyle, which is exposed. The anatomical insertion of the LCL and popliteus tendon is found (Fig. 8.5), and two anatomical tunnels usually 5–6 mm in diameter and approximately 20–25 mm in depth are created (Fig. 8.6). The two tunnels are drilled angled slightly proximal and anterior in order to avoid the intercondylar notch or any tunnels created for concomitant cruciate ligament reconstruction (Figs. 8.7 and 8.8).

A clamp is passed from the epicondyle to the fibular head beneath the IT band. The posterior band is grasped and pulled to the epicondyle, and similarly, the anterior arm is passed taking care to overlap the posterior arm always beneath the IT band, in order to recreate the same anatomical relation existing between the LCL and the popliteus tendon (Fig. 8.9). At this point, the free ends of the grafts are pulled into the femoral sockets by passing sutures that exit the medial aspect of the knee. Graft's fixation is performed first inserting a bioabsorbable screw within the fibular head, in order to avoid any slippage of the graft when fixing the two bands. Then, two bioabsorbable screws at least 1 mm larger in diameter than the tunnel size drilled are used to fix the two bands of the graft at their entry point into the femur. Alternatively, a button tying the leading sutures on the medial aspect of the knee can be used. The

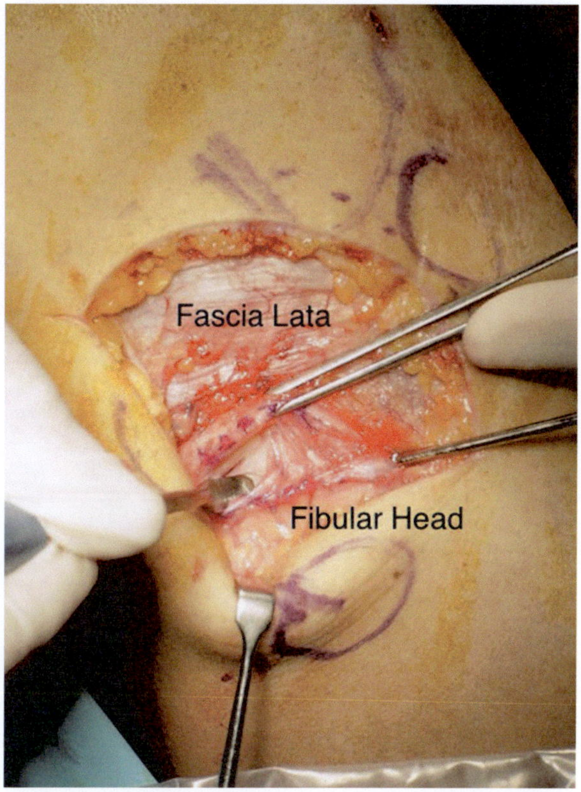

Fig. 8.4 Creation of the transfibular tunnel after dissection and protection of the space behind the fibular head

fixation of the two bands is performed with the knee flexed at 30° slightly internal rotation for the popliteus and with a valgus stress applied for the LCL.

The knee is brought through a final range of motion to ensure full motion, and stability is assessed. Any excess graft is excised, and suction drain is used only if unexpected bleeding is found at the removal of the tourniquet. Wound is closed in layers. Sterile dressings are applied, and the knee is placed into a long-leg brace in full extension with, in case of concomitant PCL reconstruction, a bolster placed beneath the tibia to prevent posterior sagging of the tibia on the femur caused by gravity. According to the concomitant surgeries performed, partial weight bearing is allowed any earlier than 3 weeks time, while usually full weight bearing is permitted 6 weeks postoperatively.

8.4 Tips and Tricks

- Always exclude any malalignment problem with a standing x-ray film and a Rosenberg view x-ray.
- Approach the surgery with a clear understanding of the degree of the lesions.

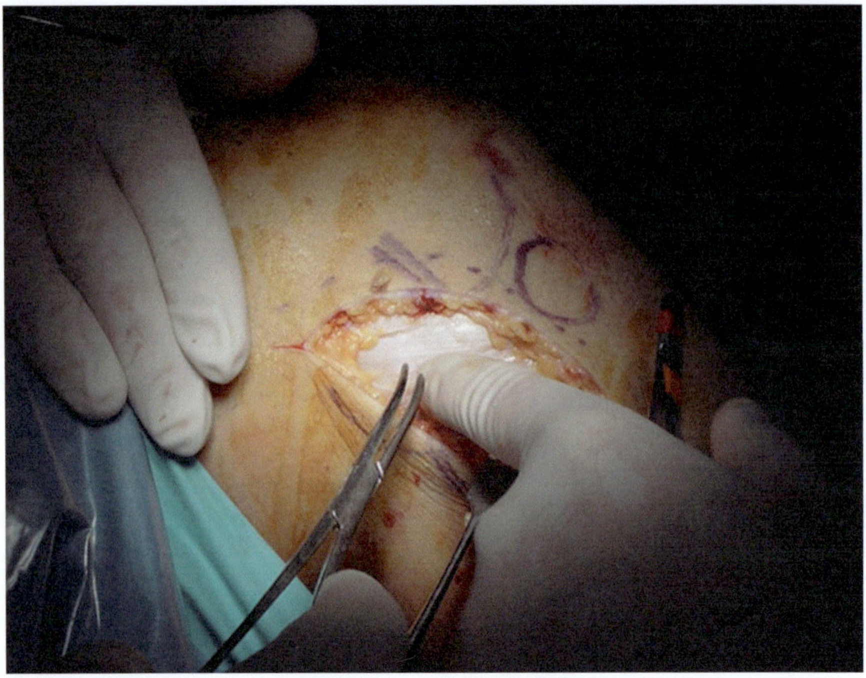

Fig. 8.5 Sometimes it is easy to find a remnant of the ligament that is used, placing the knee in a figure four position, to track the ligament up to its femoral insertion

- Get your OR familiar with your surgery.
- Position the patient in order to have full access at the knee through the entire range of motion.
- Be aware of the tourniquet time, and try to minimize the use whenever possible ACL and PCL reconstruction is performed, be aware of the tourniquet time, and try to minimize the use whenever possible.
- Do not be afraid of a large incision; the best view is the safest.
- Always identify the popliteal nerve, and protect it when drilling the fibular tunnel.
- Anatomical reconstruction needs accurate insertion exposure on the femoral epicondyle.
- Be ready to use the C-arm when creating the femoral sockets to avoid intersection with the cruciate tunnel.
- Protect your grafts after the surgery with both an appropriate brace/support and physiotherapy program.

8.5 Complications

Potential complications associated with the operative treatment of posterolateral corner injuries include peroneal nerve injury during the operative approach or reconstruction, wound problems such as infection and hematoma, hardware irritation, and knee stiffness [5].

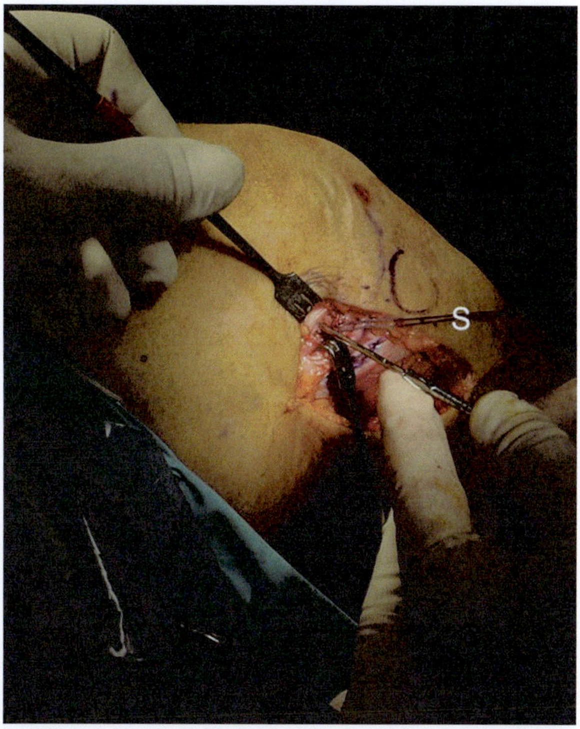

Fig. 8.6 Placement of the guide wire pro-LCL tunnel. Note the suture (S) wrapping the LCL remnant to better visualize its insertion

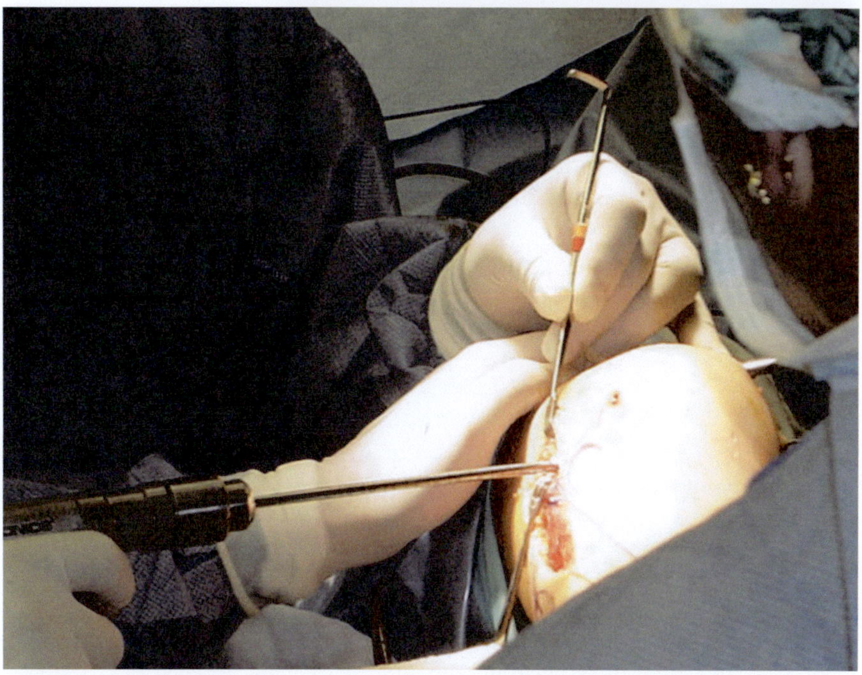

Fig. 8.7 A second tunnel is drilled to accommodate the popliteal tendon graft. The direction and inclination of these tunnels should be chosen according to the presence of other concomitant reconstructions

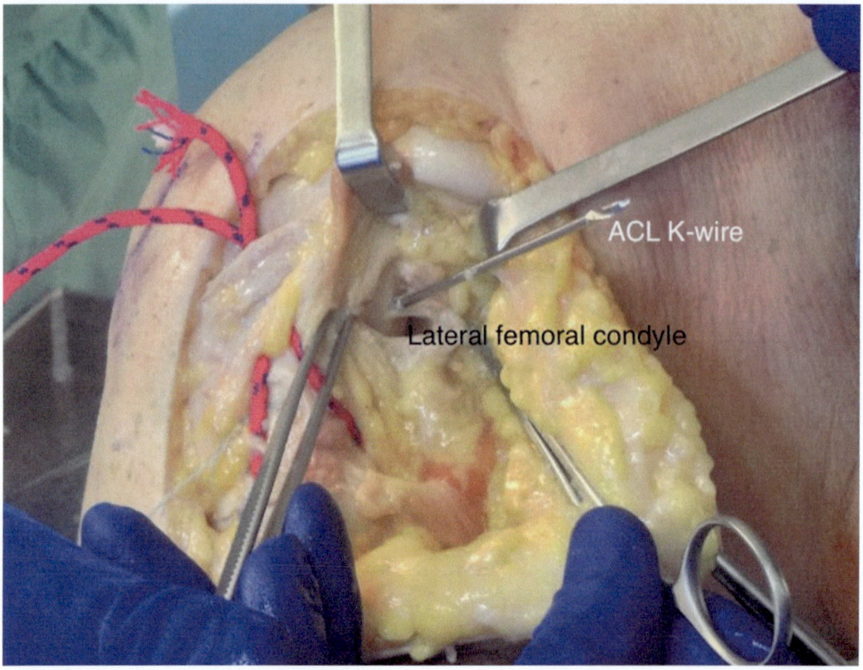

Fig. 8.8 Cadaveric specimen view showing the relationship between the ACL single bundle anatomic tunnel via AM low portal and the PLC reconstruction

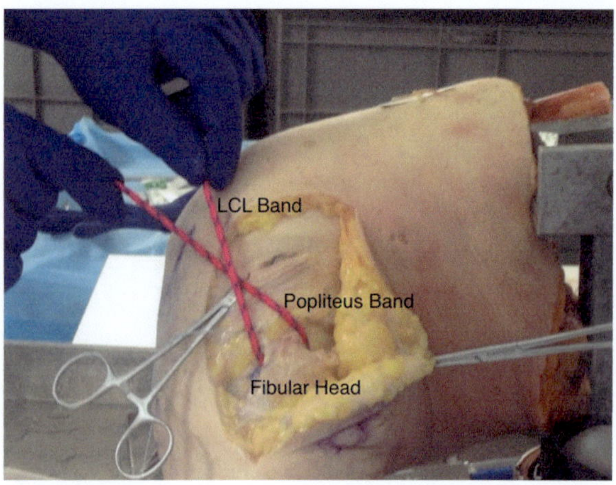

Fig. 8.9 Cadaveric specimen view of the PLC reconstruction. Please note that just for didactical purpose, the graft is placed above the fascia lata rather than below

8.6 Summary

PLC injuries are more common than expected specifically in combination with PCL tears, less frequently in association with ACL tears while isolated PLC lesion is rare. There are varying degrees of PLC injuries with respect to pathologic external tibial rotation and varus instability. Surgical treatment must address all components of the PLC (PFL, LCL, popliteus tendon) and other structural injuries. Successful PCL (and ACL) surgery depends on recognition and treatment of posterolateral corner injuries at the time of cruciate reconstructions. Despite our preferences for a fibula-based reconstruction, we recognize that one single method of reconstruction may not be suitable for all patients. Along with patient-specific factors such as the weight or the physical activity, PLC injury patterns are extremely variable. Longterm clinical studies are necessary to determine whether there is any clinical benefit of a technique over the others.

References

1. Davies H, Unwin A, Aichroth P (2004) The posterolateral corner of the knee. Anatomy, biomechanics and management of injuries. Injury 35:68–75
2. LaPrade RF, Wentorf F (2002) Diagnosis and treatment of posterolateral knee injuries. Clin Orthop Relat Res 402:110–121
3. Frank JB, Youm T, Meislin RJ, Rokito AS (2007) Posterolateral corner injuries of the knee. Bull NYU Hosp JT Dis 65:106–114
4. Cooper JM, McAndrews PT, LaPrade RF (2006) Posterolateral corner injuries of the knee: anatomy, diagnosis, and treatment. Sports Med Arthrosc 14:213–220
5. Simonian PT (2001) Operative treatment of posterolateral knee instability. Oper Tech Sports Med 9:76–83
6. Jakob RP, Hassler H, Staeubli HU (1981) Observations on rotatory instability of the lateral compartment of the knee: experimental studies on the functional anatomy and the pathomechanism of the true and the reversed pivot shift sign. Acta Orthop Scand 191:1–32
7. Clancy WG, Meister K, Craythorne CB (1995) Posterolateral corner collateral ligament reconstruction, in Jackson DW [ed]: Reconstructive Knee Surgery. New York: Raven Press, pp 143–159
8. Sidles JA, Larson RV, Garbini JL, Downey DJ, Matsen FA (1988) Ligament length relationships in the moving knee. J Orthop Res 6:593–610
9. Niki Y, Matsumoto H, Otani T, Enomoto H, Toyama Y, Suda Y (2012) A modified Larson's method of posterolateral corner reconstruction of the knee reproducing the physiological tensioning pattern of the lateral collateral and popliteofibular ligaments. Sports Med Arthrosc Rehabil Ther Technol 13:4–21
10. Veltri DM, Warren RF (1994) Anatomy, biomechanics, and physical findings in posterolateral knee instability. Clin Sports Med 13:599–614
11. Covey DC (2001) Injuries of the posterolateral corner of the knee. J Bone Joint Surg Am 83:106–118
12. Albright JP, Brown AW (1998) Management of chronic posterolateral rotatory instability of the knee: surgical technique for the posterolateral corner sling procedure. Instr Course Lect 47:369–378
13. Noyes FR, Barber-Westin DS (1995) Surgical reconstruction of severe chronic posterolateral complex injuries of the knee using allograft tissues. Am J Sports Med 23:2–12
14. LaPrade RF, Johansen S, Agel J, Risberg MA, Moksnes H, Engebretsen L (2010) Outcomes of an anatomic posterolateral knee reconstruction. J Bone Joint Surg Am 92:16–22

Surgical Approach to Posterolateral Chronic Injury

9

Evan W. James, Luke T. O'Brien, Robert F. LaPrade, and Lars Engebretsen

9.1 Preoperative Planning

The diagnosis of chronic PLC injury to the knee can be difficult and is best made using a combination of the history, physical exam, and imaging. Common mechanisms of injury include a direct blow to the anteromedial tibia in the posterolateral direction, an excessive external tibial rotation with the knee in flexion, a varus noncontact injury, and a knee hyperextension [1–4]. Special physical exam techniques are used to diagnose PLC injuries, including the external rotation recurvatum test, posterolateral drawer, dial test at 30° and 90°, varus stress test at 30°, reverse pivot shift test, and assessment for a varus thrust gait [5]. In addition, increased anterior translation on the Lachman test or increased posterior translation on the posterior drawer test may be indicative of a combined PLC injury with the respective cruciate ligament tear. In two studies with 173 total patients with PLC injuries, isolated PLC injuries represented just 28 % of cases, while combined PLC and cruciate ligament injuries were reported in 72 % of cases [6, 7].

E.W. James (✉)
Center for Outcomes-based Orthopaedic Research, Steadman Philippon Research Institute, 181 West Meadow Drive, Suite 1000, Vail, CO 81657, USA
e-mail: ejames@sprivail.org

L.T. O'Brien
Howard Head Sports Medicine, 181 West Meadow Drive, Vail, CO 81657, USA
e-mail: obrien@vvmc.com

R.F. LaPrade
The Steadman Clinic, 181 West Meadow Drive, Suite 400, Vail, CO 81657, USA
e-mail: rlaprade@thesteadmanclinic.com

L. Engebretsen
Department of Orthopaedic Surgery, Oslo University Hospital and Faculty of Medicine University of Oslo, Bergslia 22, Oslo 0870, Norway

Oslo Sports Trauma Research Center, Norwegian University of Sport Sciences, Oslo, Norway
e-mail: lars.engebretsen@medisin.uio.no

R. Rossi, F. Margheritini (eds.), *Knee Ligament Injuries*,
DOI 10.1007/978-88-470-5513-1_9, © Springer Verlag Italia 2014

Compared to minor PLC injuries, chronic complete (Grade III) PLC injuries may require surgical repair or reconstruction [8]. Before surgery, patients should undergo standing anteroposterior (AP) radiographs in full extension, lateral, sunrise, and tunnel views. Plain radiographs can help diagnose fractures, such as a fracture at the fibular head or a Segond lateral capsular avulsion fracture. Bilateral varus stress radiographs are essential to provide an objective measurement of lateral compartment gapping, which assists the clinician with differentiation of isolated FCL from complete PLC injury [5]. For an isolated FCL injury, LaPrade et al. [5] recorded a mean increase of 2.7 mm in lateral compartment gapping, while a mean increase of 4.0 mm in lateral compartment gapping was recorded for a complete (Grade III) PLC injury. In patients with chronic complete PLC injuries and concurrent genu varus, malalignment must be assessed via long leg standing radiographs and corrected first using a biplanar proximal tibial opening-wedge osteotomy. Patients should be reassessed at 6 months post surgery for residual instability before considering a PLC reconstruction [5, 9]. Arthur et al. [9] found that 38 % of patients with combined chronic complete PLC injuries and genu varus that underwent a proximal tibial osteotomy and completed a rehabilitation program did not ultimately require a PLC reconstruction. Finally, failure to correct an underlying genu varus alignment has been associated with stretching, and subsequent failure, of PLC reconstructions [10].

In patients with multiligament injuries to the PLC of the knee, Stannard et al. reported that PLC reconstructions yield significantly better outcomes than repairs [11]. In 57 knees with a minimum follow-up of 24 months, 13 of 35 repairs (37 %) resulted in failure, while 2 of 22 reconstructions (9 %) resulted in failure. Levy et al. [12] came to the same conclusion after a mean follow-up of 34 months. A total of 28 knees were studied: 10 knees underwent repair while 18 knees underwent a FCL/PLC reconstruction. Four of the 10 repairs (40 %) failed, while only 1 of the 18 reconstructions (6 %) failed ($P=0.04$). For this reason, we recommend surgical reconstruction over repair for chronic complete PLC injury. Moreover, we recommend an anatomic-based reconstruction over other nonanatomic reconstruction techniques because it has strong support biomechanically and results in significantly improved objective stability and clinical outcomes [13–19].

9.2 Surgical Technique

Anatomic-based reconstructions of the fibular collateral ligament (FCL), the popliteus tendon, and the popliteofibular ligament are our preferred techniques because they improve objective stability with varus loading and external rotation, while mimicking native anatomy (Fig. 9.1) [13–15]. Once the patient is anesthetized, a thorough examination under anesthesia is completed to assess the integrity of all ligaments. The exam findings under anesthesia can be integrated with exam findings from an earlier clinical evaluation and varus stress radiographs to render a clear understanding of all ligamentous pathologies.

After the exam under anesthesia, the knee is positioned in a leg holder at 75–80°of flexion. A standard hockey stick-shaped incision is made extending proximally along the posterior to midportion of the iliotibial band and distally at the level of

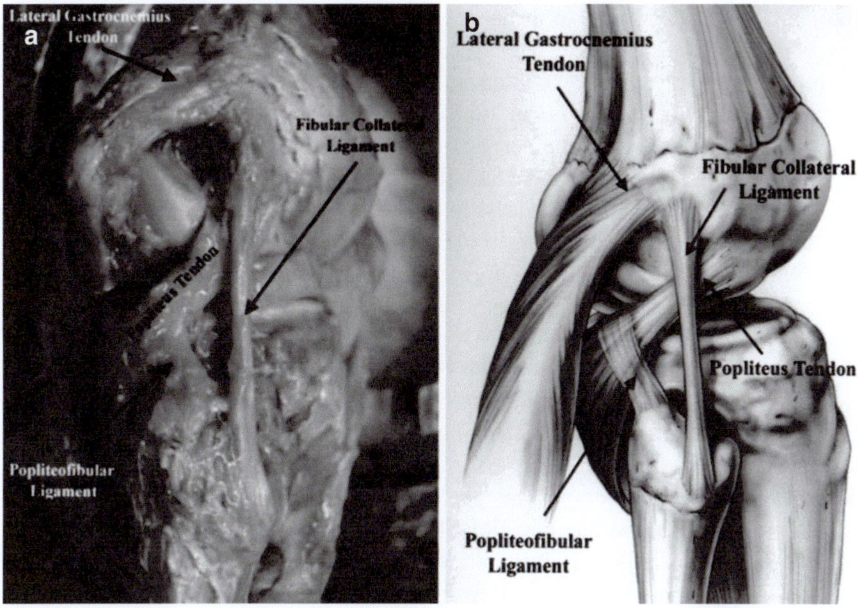

Fig. 9.1 A cadaveric photo (**a**) and illustration (**b**) depicting normal anatomy of the posterolateral corner of the knee. The popliteus tendon, popliteofibular ligament, and fibular collateral ligament comprise the main static stabilizers of the posterolateral corner (Reprinted from the *American Journal of Sports Medicine* [21])

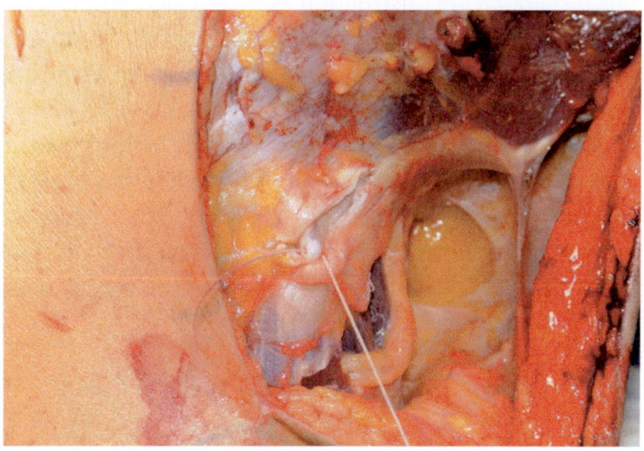

Fig. 9.2 Neurolysis of the common peroneal nerve is performed. The nerve is retracted from the surgical field as needed

Gerdy's tubercle to develop a posteriorly based skin flap [14–16, 20]. Once the superficial layer of the iliotibial band is visualized, a careful dissection is performed posteriorly using blunt dissection to isolate the long head of the biceps femoris.

Next, a peroneal neurolysis is completed to facilitate access to the posterolateral corner and to mitigate common peroneal nerve damage as a potential postoperative complication from swelling (Fig. 9.2). The common peroneal nerve is located either by palpating 2–3 cm distal to the long head of the biceps femoris or by dissecting through the fascial sheath of the peroneus longus muscle proximal to the lateral aspect of the fibular head. The nerve is carefully dissected from its connective tissue vestments for approximately 6–8 cm to allow for retraction of the nerve from the surgical field as needed for the duration of the procedure.

After the common peroneal nerve is safely identified, blunt dissection is used to enlarge the interval anterior to the lateral gastrocnemius tendon and posterior to the soleus muscle. This facilitates access to the posteromedial aspect of the fibular styloid and posterolateral tibial plateau [21]. Through this window, the musculotendinous junction of the popliteus tendon and the popliteofibular ligament, which will serve as a posterior reference point for reconstruction tunnels in the tibia and fibula, respectively, is identified.

Next, the fibular attachment of the FCL is visualized by making a small (1.5–2.0 cm long) horizontal incision 1 cm proximal to the lateral aspect of the fibular head through the anterior arm of the long head of the biceps femoris [22]. This incision allows access to the biceps bursa where the distal attachment of the FCL can readily be located. A traction stitch can be placed in the distal remnant of the FCL at this time to aid in the identification of its proximal attachment. The attachments of both the anterior aspect of the anterior arm of the long head of the biceps femoris and the FCL are carefully removed from the fibular head. A small "saddle" should be left where the FCL previously attached to the fibular head [14, 15, 21].

9.2.1 Fibular Reconstruction Tunnel

For the fibular reconstruction tunnel, a standard cannulated cruciate ligament aiming device is positioned in the posteromedial direction, entering at the attachment of the FCL on the lateral fibular head and exiting at the attachment of the popliteofibular ligament on the posteromedial fibular styloid (Fig. 9.3). Once proper alignment is achieved, a guide pin is drilled while holding a retractor posteriorly to prevent over-penetration. The position of the guide pin is assessed by palpation. Once correct positioning is confirmed, a 7-mm tunnel is reamed over the guide pin and the entry and exit sites of the tunnel are beveled with a rasp. A passing suture is then guided through the fibular tunnel to facilitate graft passage.

9.2.2 Tibial Reconstruction Tunnel

Next, Gerdy's tubercle [20] is utilized as a landmark for positioning the tibial reconstruction tunnel. All soft tissue is carefully removed distal and medial to Gerdy's tubercle to identify the flat spot where the anterior aspect of the tibial tunnel will be placed. The posterior tunnel exit point is determined by palpating deep (anterior) to the popliteus muscle at its musculotendinous junction to locate the posterior tibial popliteal sulcus. This location can also be approximated by inserting a blunt obturator into the fibular reconstruction tunnel to identify a point approximately 1 cm medial and 1 cm proximal to the obturator [14, 15, 21]. Utilizing these reference

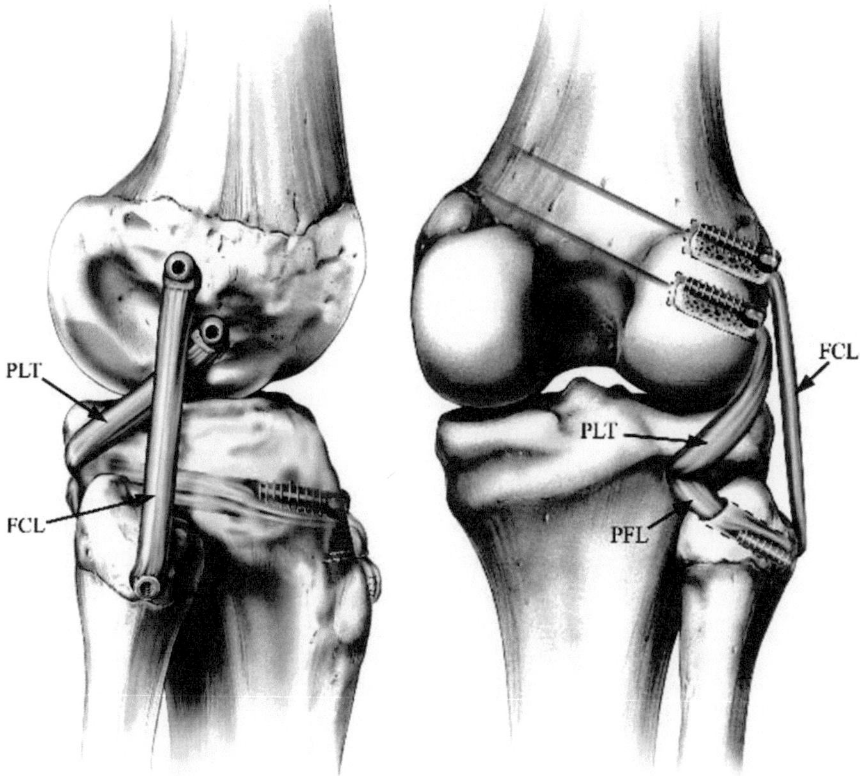

Fig. 9.3 An anatomic-based reconstruction of the posterolateral corner of the knee. *Left*, lateral view, right knee. *Right*, posterior view, right knee. Reconstructed ligaments include the main static stabilizers of the PLC: the fibular collateral ligament (*FCL*), popliteus tendon (*PLT*), and popliteofibular ligament (*PFL*) (Reprinted from the *American Journal of Sports Medicine* [14])

points, a transtibial guide pin is drilled in the anteroposterior direction from the flat spot distal and medial to Gerdy's tubercle to the musculotendinous junction of the popliteus muscle. A retractor is used to prevent over-penetration of the guide pin into the posterior neurovascular bundle. The guide pin should exit posteriorly at approximately 1 cm medial and 1 cm proximal to the obturator in the fibular reconstruction tunnel. After verifying the correct positioning of the guide pin, a 9-mm tunnel is reamed and the entry and exits of the tunnel are beveled with a rasp. Finally, a passing suture is guided through the tunnel to aid in graft passage.

9.2.3 Femoral Reconstruction Tunnels

Two femoral tunnels are required for this reconstruction. For the proximal FCL reconstruction tunnel, the proximal attachment of the FCL is located near the lateral epicondyle of the femur by applying traction to the native FCL with the traction suture. Once the attachment is found, a number 15 knife blade is used to make a small incision in the iliotibial band slightly anterior to this site. The remaining FCL is dissected from its femoral attachment. A small indentation should be left behind at the attachment site, which is used to mark the entry of the guide pin. This point is located approximately 1.4 mm proximal and 3.1 mm posterior to the lateral epicondyle. [21]. A cruciate ligament aiming device is used to pass an eyelet-tipped guide pin beginning at the femoral attachment of the FCL and traveling in the anteromedial direction. If the guide pin travels too medially, it could breach the intercondylar notch. If the guide pin travels too posteromedially, it could injure the saphenous nerve. Moreover, this orientation of the guide pin also helps to assure that the posterolateral reconstruction tunnels will not converge with an ACL or PCL graft tunnel.

Next, the intra-articular attachment of the popliteus tendon is identified on the femur by making a vertical incision in the lateral joint capsule. The location of the incision is determined either by palpating along the anterior popliteal hiatus or by measuring 2 cm anterior to the course of the fibular collateral ligament. If the popliteus tendon has not been avulsed, it can be found at the anterior fifth and proximal half of the popliteus sulcus [20, 21]. A cruciate ligament aiming device is used to pass an eyelet-tipped guide pin beginning at the attachment of the popliteus tendon in the anteromedial direction and parallel to the fibular collateral ligament guide pin. At this stage, it is critical to measure the distance between these two guide pins in order to accurately assess the restoration of native anatomy. The distance between the guide pins should be 18.5 mm, which reproduces the average distance between the center of the femoral attachments of the FCL and the popliteus tendon [14]. Finally, the guide pins are over-reamed to create two 9-mm-diameter by 25-mm-long femoral reconstruction tunnels. Any residual soft tissue is dissected away from the tunnel apertures, and passing sutures are deployed in the tunnels to facilitate graft passage.

9.2.4 Graft Preparation and Intra-articular Pathology

After completing the four reconstruction tunnels, an allograft Achilles tendon is split lengthwise. The total length of the graft should be >23 cm. The grafts are tubularized using a no. 5 suture such that each graft passes freely through the tibial and femoral reconstruction tunnels. Two 9-mm-diameter by 20-mm-long bone plugs are prepared from a calcaneus allograft to fit the femoral tunnels. Passing sutures are added to the bone and tendon grafts to help maneuver them into their respective tunnels.

At this time, any meniscal, articular cartilage, or cruciate ligament pathologies are addressed. If one or both of the cruciate ligaments require reconstruction, the tunnels are reamed and the cruciate ligament grafts are anchored in their respective femoral tunnels. The PCL graft will be fixed in its tibial tunnel prior to anchoring the reconstructed fibular collateral ligament. The ACL graft will be fixed in its tibial tunnel near the end of the procedure, due to a risk of creating a fixed external rotation deformity [23].

9.2.5 Graft Placement

After the intra-articular procedures are completed, bone plugs are inserted for the two allografts into the femoral tunnels and drawn inside by pulling the passing sutures and eyelet guide pins in the medial direction. The tendon and bone grafts are secured with a 7-mm by 20-mm cannulated interference screw. Graft fixation is tested by applying firm traction in the lateral direction.

Once both grafts are anchored securely in the femur, the popliteus tendon graft, originating at the anterior fifth of the popliteus sulcus, is passed distally through the popliteal hiatus where it will exit the knee anterior to the lateral head of the gastrocnemius. The anatomic course of the FCL is restored by passing the graft from its femoral attachment under both the superficial layers of the iliotibial band and the anterior aponeurosis of the long head of the biceps femoris. The FCL graft is then passed through the fibular tunnel in the posteromedial direction. When appropriate, the PCL graft is fixed in its tibial tunnel. The FCL graft is tensioned with the knee held in 20° flexion and a neutral tibial rotation while applying a valgus force to eliminate any potential lateral compartment gapping and secured in the fibular head tunnel with a 7-mm cannulated interference screw. Before proceeding further, the knee should be examined to ensure that all varus gapping has been eliminated by the reconstructed FCL.

Finally, both the popliteus tendon and FCL grafts are passed through the tibial tunnel in the posteroanterior direction. The remaining portion of the FCL graft, coursing medial and proximal from the posteromedial fibula to the posterolateral tibia, constitutes the reconstructed popliteofibular ligament [21]. Each graft must be checked carefully to remove any residual slack. Both grafts are tensioned simultaneously with the knee in 60° of flexion and neutral tibial rotation, and the grafts are fixed in the tibial tunnel using a 9-mm cannulated interference screw. When appropriate, the ACL graft is fixed in its tibial tunnel. The subcutaneous tissue is closed with an absorbable suture and an absorbable subcuticular stitch. An immobilizing brace should be used to prevent damage to the reconstruction as the patient awakens from anesthesia.

9.3 Postoperative Rehabilitation

Rehabilitation following PLC reconstruction follows a staged phase approach in which the first stage focuses on protecting the surgical repair and restorating normal patellofemoral and tibiofemoral range of motion (ROM). In this acute phase, patients mobilize non-weight bearing for the first 6 weeks, wear a knee immobilizer for 6 weeks, and are limited to 0–90° of knee flexion for 2 weeks before progressing to full ROM. Emphasis is placed on patellofemoral mobilization in an effort to restore patellofemoral mobility and maintain the integrity of the suprapatellar pouch and anterior interval, as well as quad activation that locks the joint in terminal extension. From weeks 7–10, the treatment emphasis remains on restoring normal ROM while progressively increasing weight-bearing tolerance. Stationary bike is initiated

Table 9.1 Postoperative restrictions

Patient remains in knee immobilizer in full knee extension at all times during the first 6 weeks postoperatively other than when working on knee range of motion (ROM) or performing quadriceps exercises
Patient with a concurrent PCL reconstruction wears the PCL Jack brace for 24 weeks, under the same parameters as above. PCL Jack brace fitted as soon as patient is able to fit into brace and tolerate its use postoperatively
Patient is to remain non-weight bearing for 6 weeks
Patient to avoid tibial external rotation and external rotation of the foot/ankle, especially in sitting for the first 4 months postoperatively
Patient to avoid hamstring exercises until 4 months postoperatively
Range of motion limited 0–90 × 2 weeks and then progressed to full range of motion
Patients with concurrent PCL reconstruction to complete ROM exercises in the prone position for 6 weeks

at this time. Once the patient is able to tolerate weight-bearing activity without negatively affecting the joint, a periodized strength program can begin. The focus of all strength programs should first be the development of a muscular endurance base upon which gains in muscular strength and power can then be made. Special focus should be placed on ensuring the correct training parameters (sets, repetitions, rest, intensity) are utilized to ensure that the desired muscular characteristic is developed. Return to running and ultimately return to sport is based on the successful completion of physical performance tests, patient reporting confidence in the knee, satisfactory stress x-ray results, and clearance by the treating physician (Table 9.1).

9.4 Surgical Outcomes

Recent outcomes studies have demonstrated improved clinical outcomes and objective stability using the anatomic-based PLC reconstruction [15]. In an in vitro biomechanical study, the 2-graft anatomic-based technique restored static varus loading and external rotation torque in knees with complete PLC injuries [14]. More recently, LaPrade et al. studied 64 Norwegian patients with chronic complete PLC injury who received either an isolated or combined posterolateral knee reconstruction. Over an average follow-up of 4.3 years, patients had an average total Cincinnati score of 65.7 points (range 20–100 points) and a significant improvement in IKDC objective scores for varus opening at 20°, external rotation at 30°, reverse pivot shift, and single leg hop [15]. These results validate the efficacy of this surgical approach for treating chronic complete posterolateral corner injuries of the knee.

9.5 Complications

As with any surgical procedure, infection can be a serious complication during the postoperative period. In addition, damage to the peroneal nerve can occur due to swelling postoperatively. The tourniquet should be let down prior to closing the surgical incision in order to cauterize bleeding vessels, as formation of a hematoma at the fibular neck has been reported to cause common peroneal nerve palsy [24]. Signs of peroneal nerve damage include numbness in the first foot web space, numbness along the dorsum of the foot, and loss of plantar dorsiflexion, foot eversion, and great toe extensions. These deficits classically manifest as a foot drop and a steppage gait. Other signs of postsurgical complications include lack of full knee extension, recurrent knee instability, knee catching or locking, signs of a deep vein thrombosis such as calf tenderness, and increased knee effusion with activity.

Conclusions

Chronic PLC injuries of the knee are no longer the enigma they were 20 years ago. Anatomic and biomechanical studies of the posterolateral corner of the knee have allowed for the development of biomechanically validated reconstructions that reproduce the native structure and function of the injured static stabilizers. The technique outlined in this chapter has also been validated clinically to improve clinical outcomes and objective stability. Additional follow-up studies are needed to track the long-term effectiveness of this anatomic-based surgical reconstruction with the goal of improving recovery times and maximizing restoration of function.

References

1. Fleming RE Jr, Blatz DJ, McCarroll JR (1981) Posterior problems in the knee: posterior cruciate insufficiency and posterolateral rotatory insufficiency. Am J Sports Med 9:107–113
2. Fornalski S, McGarry MH, Csintalan RP et al (2008) Biomechanical and anatomical assessment after knee hyperextension injury. Am J Sports Med 36:80–84
3. LaPrade RF, Hamilton CD, Engebretsen L (1997) Treatment of acute and chronic combined anterior cruciate ligament and posterolateral knee ligament injuries. Sports Med Arthrosc Rev 5:91–99
4. LaPrade RF, Muench C, Wentorf FA et al (2002) The effect of injury to the posterolateral structures of the knee on force in a posterior cruciate ligament graft: a biomechanical study. Am J Sports Med 30:233–238
5. LaPrade RF, Engebretsen L, Johansen S (2008) The effect of a proximal tibial medial opening wedge osteotomy on posterolateral knee instability; a biomechanical study. Am J Sports Med 36:956–960
6. Geeslin AG, LaPrade RF (2010) Location of bone bruises and other osseous injuries associated with acute grade III isolated and combined posterolateral knee injuries. Am J Sports Med 38:2502–2508
7. LaPrade RF, Terry GC (1997) Injuries to the posterolateral aspect of the knee: association of anatomic injury patterns with clinical instability. Am J Sports Med 25:433–438
8. Kannus P (1989) Nonoperative treatment of grade II and III sprains of the lateral ligament compartment of the knee. Am J Sports Med 17:85–88
9. Arthur A, LaPrade RF, Agel J (2007) Proximal tibial opening wedge osteotomy as the initial treatment for chronic posterolateral corner deficiency in the varus knee: a prospective clinical study. Am J Sports Med 35:1844–1850
10. Noyes FR, Barber-Westin SD (1996) Surgical restoration to treat chronic deficiency of the posterolateral complex and cruciate ligaments of the knee joint. Am J Sports Med 28:282–296

11. Stannard JP, Brown SL, Farris RC et al (2005) The posterolateral corner of the knee: repair versus reconstruction. Am J Sports Med 33:881–888
12. Levy BA, Dajani KA, Morgan JA (2010) Repair versus reconstruction of the fibular collateral ligament and posterolateral corner in the multiligament-injured knee. Am J Sports Med 38:804–809
13. Coobs BR, LaPrade RF, Griffith CJ et al (2007) Biomechanical analysis of an isolated fibular (lateral) collateral ligament reconstruction using an autogenous semitendinosus graft. Am J Sports Med 35:1521–1527
14. LaPrade RF, Johansen S, Wentorf FA et al (2004) An analysis of an anatomical posterolateral knee reconstruction: an in vitro biomechanical study and development of a surgical technique. Am J Sports Med 32:1405–1414
15. LaPrade RF, Johansen S, Agel J et al (2010) Outcomes of an anatomic posterolateral knee reconstruction. J Bone Joint Surg Am 92:16–22
16. LaPrade RF, Johansen S, Engebretsen L (2011) Outcomes of an anatomic posterolateral knee reconstruction: surgical technique. J Bone Joint Surg Am 93(Suppl 1):10–20
17. Lee MC, Park YK, Lee SH et al (2003) Posterolateral reconstruction using split Achilles tendon allograft. Arthroscopy 19:1043–1049
18. Sekiya JK, Kurtz CA (2005) Posterolateral corner reconstruction of the knee: surgical technique utilizing a bifid Achilles tendon allograft and a double femoral tunnel. Arthroscopy 21:1400.e1–1400.e5
19. Yoon KH, Bae DK, Ha JH et al (2006) Anatomic reconstructive surgery for posterolateral instability of the knee. Arthroscopy 22:159–165
20. Terry GC, LaPrade RF (1996) The posterolateral aspect of the knee: anatomy and surgical approach. Am J Sports Med 24:732–739
21. LaPrade RF, Ly TV, Wentorf FA et al (2003) The posterolateral attachments of the knee: a quantitative and qualitative morphologic analysis of the fibular collateral ligament, popliteus tendon, popliteofibular ligament, and lateral gastrocnemius tendon. Am J Sports Med 31:854–860
22. LaPrade RF, Hamilton CD (1997) The fibular collateral ligament-biceps femoris bursa. An anatomic study. Am J Sports Med 25:439–443
23. Wentorf FA, LaPrade RF, Lewis JL et al (2002) The influence of the integrity of posterolateral structures on tibiofemoral orientation when an anterior cruciate ligament graft is tensioned. Am J Sports Med 20:796–799
24. Girolami M, Galletti S, Montanari G, Mignani G, Schuh R, Ellis S, Di Motta D, D'Apote G, Bevoni R (2013) Common Peroneal Nerve Palsy due to Hematoma at the Fibular Neck. J Knee Surg 26(Suppl 1):S132–135.

HTO and Peripheral Instability

10

Federica Rosso, Salvatore Bisicchia,
and Annunziato Amendola

10.1 Limb Alignment and Tibial Slope

Normal anatomic lower limb alignment on the coronal plane is somewhat variable but falls within 5° and 7° of valgus [1–7]. Similarly, a wide range of values of medial and lateral tibial slope are reported in literature because different radiographic techniques have been described [8–10]. In the normal knee, the medial posterior tibial slope is usually 6–11° and the lateral one is 9–11° [10–16]. Meniscal or cartilage loss and ligament attenuation lead to an increased deformity over time.

Individuals with a *preexisting malalignment* of the lower limb and a significant knee ligamentous injury may not do well with an isolated ligamentous reconstruction. The neuromuscular or proprioceptive control of the joint provided by the soft tissue structures may be lost when ligamentous disruption occurs, resulting in increased malalignment and subjective instability [17]. In this scenario realignment surgery augments ligamentous reconstruction and improves overall joint function and stability.

Alignment in the sagittal plane can indeed affect knee stability. Increased tibial slope causes increased anterior tibial translation and the tendency of the femur to slide posteriorly along the tibial slope [18, 19]. In cases of anterior cruciate ligament (ACL) deficiency, anterior tibial translation can be magnified in the presence of an increased slope. Posterior cruciate ligament (PCL)-deficient knees, on the other hand, are stabilized by increasing tibial slope, reducing the posterior translation [20].

F. Rosso, MD
Department of Orthopaedic and Traumatology, University of Study of Turin,
AO Mauriziano Umberto I, Largo Turati 62, Turin 10125, Italy

S. Bisicchia, MD
Department of Orthopaedic Surgery, University of Rome "Tor Vergata",
Viale Oxford 81, Rome 00133, Italy

A. Amendola, MD (✉)
Department of Orthopaedic Surgery, UI Sports Medicine,
University of Iowa Hospitals and Clinics, 200 Hawkins Drive, Iowa City, IA 52242, USA
e-mail: ned-amendola@uiowa.edu

R. Rossi, F. Margheritini (eds.), *Knee Ligament Injuries*,
DOI 10.1007/978-88-470-5513-1_10, © Springer Verlag Italia 2014

10.1.1 Alignment and Instability

10.1.1.1 Triple Varus Knee

Noyes described the mechanism associating the tibiofemoral alignment with ligament instability: this deformity was called the *triple varus knee* [21]. In the ACL-deficient knee, preexisting varus malalignment can cause progressive medial compartment degeneration or medial meniscus injury. This may lead to medial compartment narrowing, and the weight-bearing axis may shift medially, resulting in a primary varus. With progressive narrowing, posterolateral structures become lax, leading to a double varus. If the malalignment becomes more chronic, the overload on the posterolateral structures may lead to hyperextension recurvatum deformity, referred as triple varus [22–24]. In this scenario an ACL reconstruction alone will decrease the anterior tibial translation, without correcting the varus deformity, leading to continuous stress on the graft and potential increasing laxity.

Acute injury to the posterolateral complex in combination with preexisting varus simulates a triple varus knee, and PCL injury can increase the hyperextension deformity.

10.1.1.2 Pure Varus or Valgus Malalignment

Pure varus malalignment can develop after an isolated injury to the lateral collateral ligament, developing a varus thrust causing pain and symptomatic instability [25].

On the contrary static valgus laxities due to medial side injuries have not been reported. However, they can occur in limbs with preexisting valgus deformity and medial side injury without treatment [26].

10.1.1.3 Unicompartmental Degeneration with Malalignment

In the presence of meniscal or cartilage injuries, a chronic ligamentous laxity may lead to malalignment and unicompartmental overload and degeneration [27]. These conditions are most commonly associated with chronic PCL or ACL deficiency. In this scenario an osteotomy can be indicated to unload the involved compartment, reduce pain, and improve the stability or thrust. In these cases, where additional ligament surgery may be necessary, reconstruction can be performed in a concomitant or staged manner [28].

10.2 Indication and Rationale for HTO in Peripheral Instability

In has been demonstrated that high tibial osteotomy (HTO) can modify not only the coronal but also the sagittal plane of the knee [29, 30]. Some authors [31, 32] demonstrated that a lateral closing-wedge HTO causes a decrease in *posterior tibial slope* with posterior translation of the tibia, resulting in stabilization of a knee with anterior instability. On the contrary, a medial opening-wedge HTO increases the posterior tibial slope causing an anterior translation of the tibia, resulting in a stabilization of a knee with posterior instability [8, 20] (Fig. 10.1). In particular, Griffin et al. [33] reported that, after an anterior opening-wedge HTO, the posterior tibial

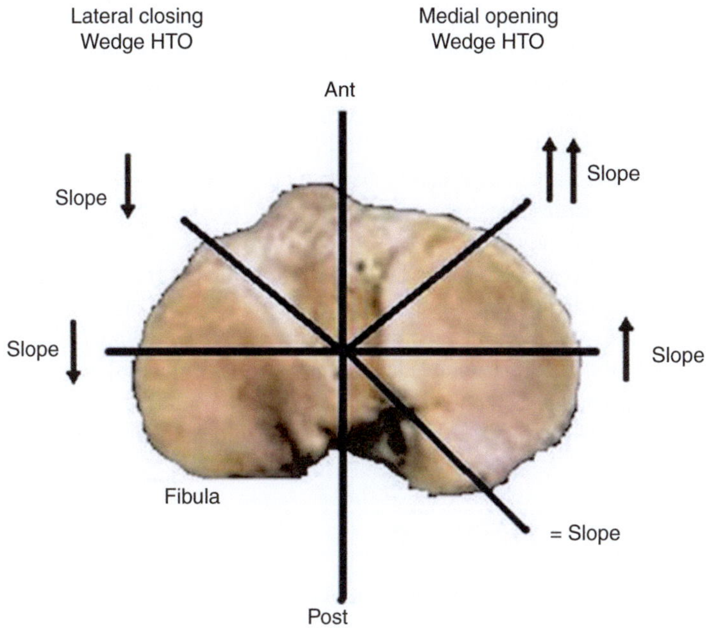

Fig. 10.1 Relationship between tibial slope and kind and site of osteotomy

slope increased from 8.8° ± 1.8° to 13.2° ± 2.1°, causing an anterior translation of the tibia of 3.6 ± 1.4 mm compared with the starting position. Furthermore, forces on PCL decreased from 34 ± 14 N to 19 ± 15 N with the knee flexed at 30° and from 36 ± 29 N to 22 ± 11 N with the knee flexed at 90°.

For these reasons, HTO may be indicated in patients who have posterolateral laxity and varus hyperextension thrust, ACL deficiency and varus thrust, or alignment and combined ligamentous laxity with varus or posterolateral thrust. In these patients poor results with the ligamentous reconstructive surgery alone have been reported, and soft tissue surgery should not be performed until the alignment has been corrected [34].

In general, our approach is to perform HTO first since in most of the cases with posterolateral or lateral instability, correcting the alignment will correct the instability symptoms. Normally, after 6–8 months from the realignment surgery, we evaluate the patient, and if there are still symptoms of instability, the ligamentous surgery can be performed. On the contrary, in the case of combined ACL deficiency and malalignment in a young patient, we would perform a concurrent ACL reconstruction and HTO [35].

10.3 Operative Techniques

Although different techniques are available to correct a varus alignment, the opening-wedge HTO is preferred by the majority of the surgeons. Its *advantages* include multiplanar correction, avoidance of the proximal tibiofibular joint and peroneal nerve, and possible intraoperative adjustment. Furthermore, if a collateral ligament laxity is present, it can be improved by distraction from the opening wedge.

Disadvantages include the possible need for a bone graft and difficult correction of severe deformity. However, in the unstable knee the correction required is often from 5° to 15°, so the opening-wedge HTO is acceptable. The lateral closing-wedge HTO decreases the tibial slope, and it can be used to correct chronic anterior instabilities. The static valgus laxities due to medial side injuries can occur in limbs with preexisting valgus deformity and medial injuries without proper treatment, but they are much rarer. To produce varus effect, either a closing-wedge medial HTO or a distal femoral osteotomy (DFO) can be used. Because of the concern of joint obliquity, the closing-wedge medial HTO is recommended by few authors [26], while most of the literature recommends a DFO, but it is not able to correct the tibial slope [36]. For these reasons and because this chapter is focused on HTO and peripheral instabilities only, the surgical technique for a medial opening-wedge HTO will be explained.

10.3.1 Preoperative Planning

For a correct preoperative planning of an HTO, *plain radiographs* are mandatory. Bilateral weight-bearing anteroposterior views in full extension, bilateral weight-bearing posteroanterior tunnel views at 30° of flexion, and anteroposterior, lateral, and skyline views are recommended to appreciate the lower limb alignment and the amount of arthrosis. Furthermore a single-leg weight-bearing anteroposterior view is also obtained to appreciate the severity of varus thrust [37].

Supine X-rays are important to eliminate the added varus due to deficiency of the lateral and/or posterolateral structures and to evaluate the real amount of correction to perform. Several stress radiographs have been described to evaluate translation of the tibia compared to the contralateral side [38]. Magnetic resonance imaging can be useful to assess the presence of cartilage damages or meniscal and ligamentous injuries, and specific sequences are required to better visualize the posterolateral corner [39]. We calculate the required correction using the method described by Dugdale et al. [40]. HTO is planned so to place the weight-bearing axis falling at 62.5 % across the width of the tibial plateau from medial to lateral. If there is no medial space narrowing, this line can also be positioned in the middle of the tibial plateau. In the presence of PCL deficiency, HTO should be planned to increase the posterior tibial slope in the sagittal plane reducing the posterior subluxation of the tibia relatively to the femur. In this scenario, the wedge needs to be positioned anteromedially. On the other hand, if a chronic ACL deficiency is associated with the malalignment, the wedge needs to be as far posterior as possible [41] (Fig. 10.2).

10.3.2 Surgical Technique

All patients routinely receive intravenous antibiotics preoperatively; either general or spinal anesthesia is used.

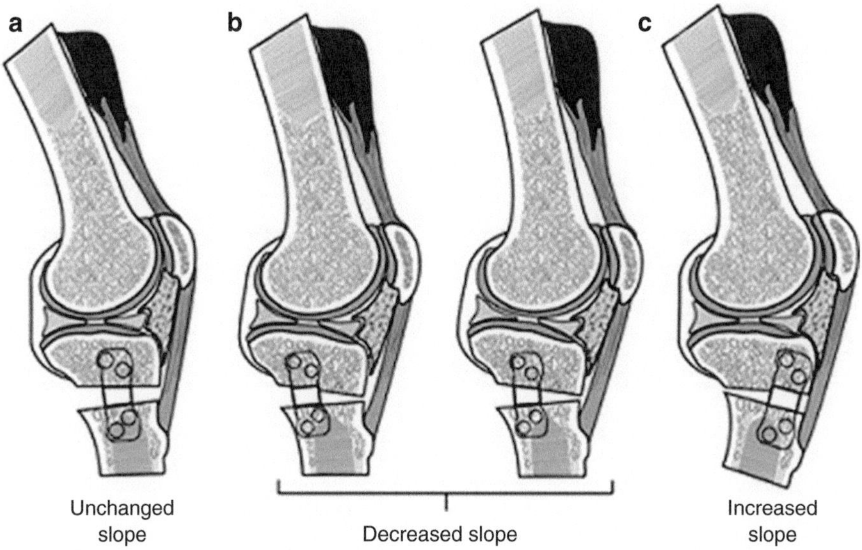

Fig. 10.2 Demonstration of the relationship between wedge position and tibial slope. (**a**) Medial placement of the wedge resulting in no alterations of the tibial slope. (**b**) Posteromedial placement of the wedge resulting in decreased tibial slope, useful in ACL-deficient knees. (**c**) Anteromedial placement of the wedge resulting in increased tibial slope, useful in PCL-deficient knees (© 2011 American Academy of Orthopaedic Surgeons. Reprinted from Rossi et al. [42] with permission)

10.3.2.1 Opening-Wedge Medial HTO Stabilized with a Plate and Screws

The patient is positioned supine, the lower limb is prepared and draped, and a tourniquet is positioned on the thigh. *Arthroscopy* should be performed in patients to confirm the indication and evaluate the intra-articular status; after this step the tourniquet is inflated. An anteromedial vertical incision is performed midway between the medial border of the tubercle and the posterior border of the tibia, just below the pes anserinus and 1 cm below the joint line. The sartorial fascia is elevated to visualize the hamstring and the superficial medial collateral ligament (MCL), and a blunt retractor is placed posteriorly to protect both these structures and the neurovascular ones. The patellar tendon is exposed and protected. Under fluoroscopic control, a *guide wire* is positioned from medial to lateral, at the level of the superior aspect of the tibial tubercle, anteromedially, arriving 1 cm below the joint line (Fig. 10.3a). A cortical osteotomy is performed using and oscillating saw, inferiorly to the guide wire to prevent superior migration and intra-articular fractures, and it is continued with an osteotome under fluoroscopic control. Once the *osteotomy* is completed, the medial opening is created using an apposite wedge placed to the planned depth (Fig. 10.3b). A wedge placed anteriorly causes an increase of the tibial slope, while, if the wedge is placed posteriorly, a slight decrease of the tibial slope is achieved [41]. Anterior and posterior gaps are then measured in order to calculate the amount of slope modification as described by Noyes et al. [30]: if the anteromedial gap is

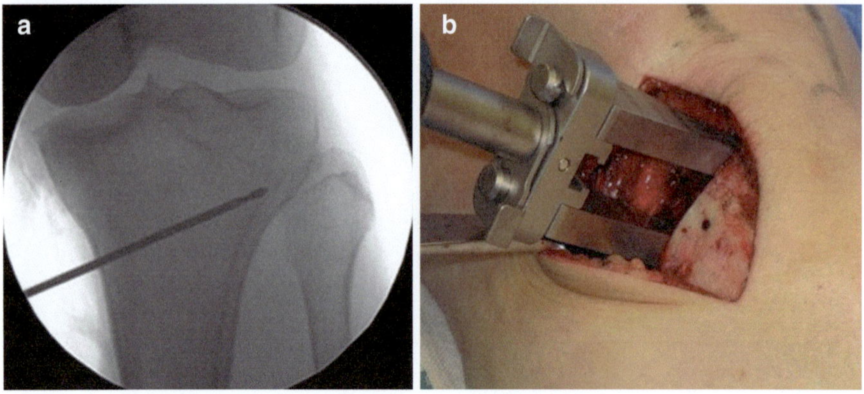

Fig. 10.3 (**a**) A guide wire is placed from the superior aspect of the tibial tubercle to about 1 cm below the lateral joint line. (**b**) Cortical osteotomy is performed with an oscillating saw and continued with osteotomes just behind the guide wire. Once the osteotomy is completed, the medial opening is created using a dedicated wedge placed to the planned depth

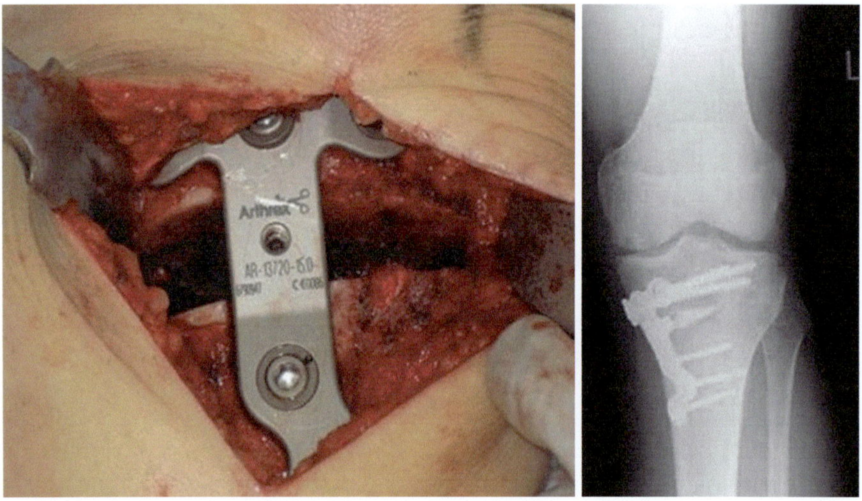

Fig. 10.4 The osteotomy is stabilized with the plate (Arthrex, Naples, Florida)

half of the posteromedial, the tibial slope will not change; otherwise for each 1 mm of increase in the anterior gap, the posterior slope will increase by 2°. Furthermore, if the anterior gap is greater than 1 cm, a tibial tubercle osteotomy is recommended in order to avoid patella infera. The lower limb alignment is checked under fluoroscopic control, and the gap is filled with either autograft, allograft, or synthetic bone. Finally, the osteotomy is stabilized using a contour lock or 4-hole plate (Arthrex, Naples, FL, USA) with 6.5 mm cancellous screws proximally and 4.5 mm cortical screws distally (Fig. 10.4). The final result is checked under fluoroscopic control, the tourniquet is deflated, and the wound is closed in a standard fashion.

With small corrections, a *4-hole plate* will be satisfactory, but for large corrections and biplanar correction, the *contour lock plate* is preferred.

10.3.2.2 Opening-Wedge Medial HTO with the iBalance System

Although good long-term results are reported with opening-wedge HTO, it remains a challenging procedure with some intraoperative risks like neurovascular injury, fracture of the lateral cortical hinge or fracture into the lateral tibial plateau and resultant osteotomy instability, loss of correction, and delayed/nonunion of the osteotomy. To make the medial opening-wedge HTO a more reproducible procedure with less risk of complications, the *iBalance™ HTO system* (Arthrex, Naples, FL) was developed. It includes an instrumentation with a neurovascular blunt retractor, a patellar retractor, an alignment handle, and a new cutting guide. With this system the surgeon is able to reduce the risk of fracture by hinging on a predrilled hole to allow dissipation of forces laterally; besides the alignment handle allows to easily check the correction both on the sagittal and coronal plane. The novel implant is made of *polyetheretherketone* (PEEK), a new radiolucent and bio-inert material which is already used in different orthopedic implants [43]. In literature this system has been described to be safe and with some advantages like the protection of the neurovascular bundle, a low profile nature of the implant reducing soft tissue irritation, and the ability to maintain the alignment in both the coronal and sagittal planes [44].

The approach is the same we described in the above section. After the detachment of the medial collateral ligament and the exposition of the patellar tendon, the *alignment handle* with the keyhole guide is positioned with the patellar retractor, and the alignment is checked with the C-arm on both the sagittal and coronal plane. The *biplanar alignment bars* should be positioned on the joint line on the anteroposterior view, and the two bars should appear as a single one on the lateral view. Once the correct alignment in both planes is obtained, the keyhole guide is fixed with pins and the alignment handle is removed. At this point a *keyhole reamer* is used to drill two holes to allow dissipation of forces laterally and to accommodate the plate. Now the cutting guide and the neurovascular blunt retractor are assembled to the system. The cut is performed and the system is removed; now the *opening jack paddles* are inserted into the osteotomy, and the correction is obtained slowly opening the jack by turning the turn key handle. Once the correction is obtained, the iBalance™ PEEK implant can be positioned; the gap is filled with autologous bone graft from the drilled holes and bone substitute can be used. The PEEK plate is fixed with two cancellous anchors (screws) proximally and two cortical anchors distally. Figure 10.5 shows few steps of this technique.

10.3.2.3 Opening Medial HTO Stabilized with External Fixator

We normally use a circular external fixator (Taylor Spatial Frame™, Smith and Nephew) with gradual correction only if the deformity is large, usually greater than 17.5°. In these cases, the fixator is assembled preoperatively using three rings 4 cm larger than the diameter of the leg. Preoperatively the correction is calculated in each plane and if any length needs to be adjusted, but then this is confirmed after application of the fixator postoperatively. The first ring is positioned

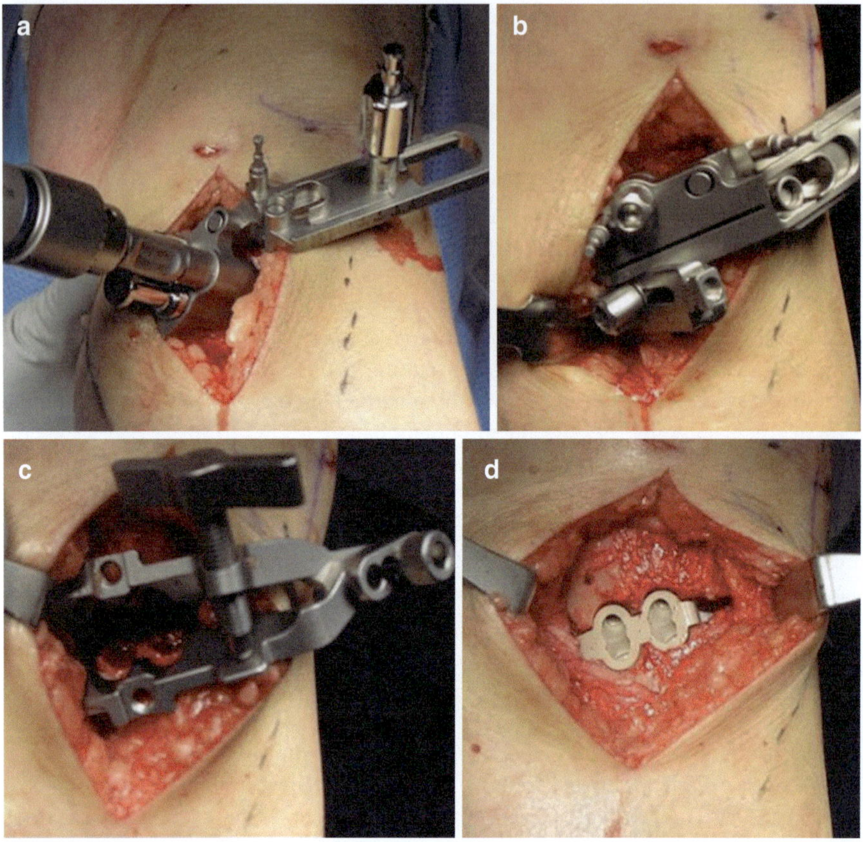

Fig. 10.5 iBalance technique. (**a**) The keyhole reamer drilling the two holes. (**b**) The cutting guide. (**c**) The opening jack paddles are inserted into the osteotomy; to open the osteotomy turn the key handle until the planned correction angle is noted on the correction guide. (**d**) The iBalance PEEK plate is positioned and stabilized with two cancellous anchors proximally and two cortical anchors distally

at the level of the fibular head and the second below the tibial tubercle, and they are joined by the six correction rods. The third ring is preset approximately 5 cm distal to the second one using four tethered rods. The proximal ring is placed parallel to the tibial articular surface in both the coronal and sagittal planes. The two distal rings are aligned to the tibial shaft, and the deformity to be corrected is between the first and second ring. The apparatus is then sterilized, the lower limb is prepared, and the tourniquet is inflated. A 3-cm incision is made 10 cm below the fibular head posterolaterally, the plane between soleus and peronei is developed, and an oblique fibular osteotomy is performed. The external fixator is then applied to the leg. The first ring is secured using two wires and one half-pin across the tibia, and the second ring is then secured with one wire and one half-pin across the tibia (to avoid the peroneal branches, the pins should be placed more laterally

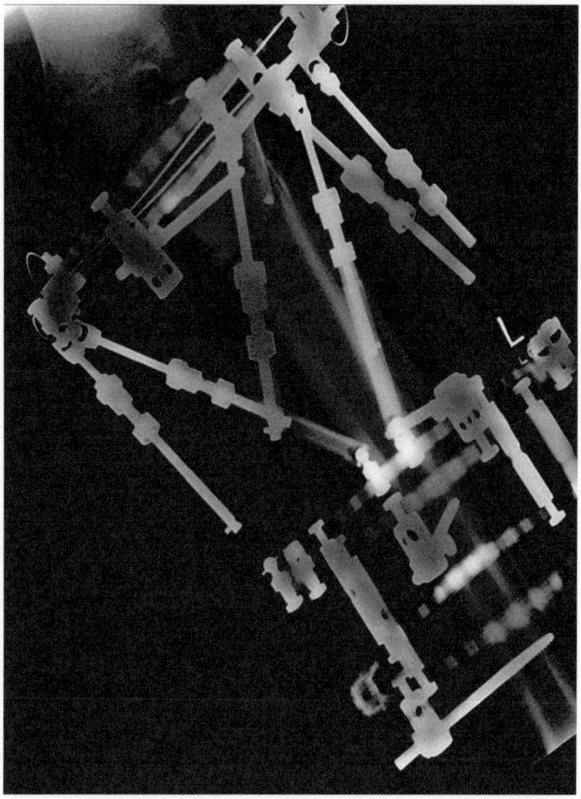

Fig. 10.6 Radiographic picture showing an external fixator used for an osteotomy

than medially). The third ring is stabilized with two wires passing across the tibia. At this point a 1.5-cm incision is performed anteriorly just distal to the tibial tubercle, the periosteum is elevated, and a tibial osteotomy is performed (Fig. 10.6). Some correction can be performed during the surgery to ensure the osteotomy will correct, and then it can be gradually done beginning 7–10 days postoperatively (callotasis).

10.3.3 Postoperative Protocol

If a plate is used to stabilize the osteotomy, the patient will be toe-touch weight bearing for 6 weeks. In this period the knee will be protected into an articulated brace locked in extension during ambulation. After 6 weeks X-rays are performed, and if there are no problems, the patient is encouraged to increase weight bearing and discontinue the crutches and the brace progressively until 10–12 weeks, when another X-ray is recommended to ensure healing. If a circular external fixator is used, the patient is allowed partial weight bearing immediately without any brace.

10.4 Outcomes

In literature good results are reported regarding HTO alone or combined with ligamentous reconstructions. In cases of lower limb malalignment, in both the coronal and sagittal planes, an opening-wedge HTO can restore the alignment and resolve symptomatic posterior instability. Some authors reported good results using either a closing-wedge or an opening-wedge HTO in a varus ACL-deficient knee; furthermore, HTO associated with ACL reconstruction showed good results in young and active patients [8, 19, 23, 31, 45, 46]. Noyes et al. [23] reported the results in 23 double varus and in 18 triple varus knees, all associated with ACL deficiency. In all the patients they performed a lateral closing-wedge HTO with good results in almost 83 % of the patients. Dejour et al. [47] reported on 50 ACL-deficient knees with acquired varus deformity in which they performed an HTO with ACL reconstruction and extra-articular procedures if necessary. At a mean follow-up of 43 months, they reported 91 % of satisfactory results. Fowler et al. [45] reported on 7 ACL-deficient knees with varus alignment or thrust and medial osteoarthritis in which they performed an isolated HTO with significant improvement of stability and alignment in all the cases. Boss et al. [48] performed 24 lateral closing-wedge and 3 medial opening-wedge HTOs in 27 patients with an ACL reconstruction, and they reported 75 % of good results.

There are a few papers reporting on the *results* of medial opening-wedge osteotomies in patients with posterolateral instabilities. Naudie et al. [28] reported on 17 symptomatic posterolateral-deficient knees with hyperextension or varus thrust, in which a medial opening-wedge HTO with correction on the tibial slope was performed. Their results were satisfactory in 16/17 patients, with one case of delayed union and one of displaced tibial tubercle osteotomy. Arthur et al. [49] performed 8 isolated medial opening-wedge HTOs and 13 combined with delayed ligamentous reconstruction in 21 patients with posterolateral corner deficiency and genu varum. They concluded that poorer results can be obtained when a delayed ligamentous surgery is needed.

Possible complications from this surgery are related not only to the osteotomy but, in the majority of the cases, to an undercorrection on both coronal and sagittal planes. According to Noyes et al. [23], we suggest that in the presence of narrowing of the medial compartment, the mechanical axis should be placed laterally to the center of the knee, avoiding early recurrence of the deformity on the coronal plane. For the sagittal plane, the most common complication is to have too much opening anteriorly, resulting in lack of extension and patella baja. Disadvantages in using an opening-wedge HTO are an unstable construct, implant failure, delayed union, and nonunions. On the other hand, potential disadvantages using an external fixator are discomfort for the patient and pin tract infection, and because the external fixator is not rigid, a loss of correction may occur. For these reasons we prefer to perform an HTO reserving the external fixation only if a correction more than 17.5° is needed.

Although the experience of using osteotomy in the presence of knee instability is limited, the results are encouraging in the chronic unstable knee. Longer follow-up studies are necessary before definitive recommendations can be made regarding the long-term outcome and function of these procedures.

References

1. Kapandji IA (1970) The physiology of the joints: annotated diagrams of the mechanics of the human joints. E. & S. Livingstone, London
2. Chao EY (1976) The biomechanics of total joint replacement surgery. Geriatrics 31:48–57
3. Krackow KA (1983) Approaches to planning lower extremity alignment for total knee arthroplasty and osteotomy about the knee. Adv Orthop Surg 7:69
4. Moreland JR, Bassett LW, Hanker GJ (1987) Radiographic analysis of the axial alignment of the lower extremity. J Bone Joint Surg Am 69:745–749
5. Hsu RW, Himeno S, Coventry MB, Chao EY (1990) Normal axial alignment of the lower extremity and load-bearing distribution at the knee. Clin Orthop Relat Res 255:215–227
6. Paley D, Tetsworth K (1992) Mechanical axis deviation of the lower limbs. Preoperative planning of uniapical angular deformities of the tibia or femur. Clin Orthop Relat Res 1:48–64
7. Hungerford DS (1995) Alignment in total knee replacement. Instr Course Lect 44:455–468
8. Dejour H, Bonnin M (1994) Tibial translation after anterior cruciate ligament rupture. Two radiological tests compared. J Bone Joint Surg Br 76:745–749
9. Moore TM, Harvey JP Jr (1974) Roentgenographic measurement of tibial-plateau depression due to fracture. J Bone Joint Surg Am 56:155–160
10. Brazier J, Migaud H, Gougeon F, Cotten A, Fontaine C, Duquennoy A (1996) Evaluation of methods for radiographic measurement of the tibial slope. A study of 83 healthy knee. Rev Chir Orthop Reparatrice Appar Mot 82:195–200
11. Lecuire F, Lerat JL, Bousquet G, Dejour H, Trillat A (1980) The treatment of genu recurvatum. Rev Chir Orthop Reparatrice Appar Mot 66:95–103
12. Paley D, Herzenberg JE, Tetsworth K, McKie J, Bhave A (1994) Deformity planning for frontal and sagittal plane corrective osteotomies. Orthop Clin North Am 25:425–465
13. Insall JN (1993) Total knee arthroplasty in rheumatoid arthritis. Ryumachi 33:472
14. Matsuda S, Miura H, Nagamine R, Urabe K, Ikenoue T, Okazaki K, Iwamoto Y (1999) Posterior tibial slope in the normal and varus knee. Am J Knee Surg 12:165–168
15. Chiu KY, Zhang SD, Zhang GH (2000) Posterior slope of tibial plateau in Chinese. J Arthroplasty 15:224–227
16. Genin P, Weill G, Julliard R (1993) The tibial slope. Proposal for a measurement method. J Radiol 74:27–33
17. Lephart SM, Pincivero DM, Rozzi SL (1998) Proprioception of the ankle and knee. Sports Med 25:149–155
18. Dejour H, Walch G, Chambat P (1988) Active subluxation in extension: a new concept of study of the ACL-deficient knee. Am J Knee Surg 1:204–211
19. Dejour H, Neyret P, Bonnin M (1994) Instability and osteoarthritis in knee surgery. In: Knee surgery. Williams & Wilkins, Baltimore, pp 859–875
20. Giffin JR, Stabile KJ, Zantop T, Vogrin TM, Woo SL, Harner CD (2007) Importance of tibial slope for stability of the posterior cruciate ligament deficient knee. Am J Sports Med 35(9):1443–1449
21. Noyes FR, Simon R (1194) The role of high tibial osteotomy in the anterior cruciate ligament-deficient knee. In: DeLee JC, Drez D (eds) Orthopaedic sports medicine. Principles and practice. WB Saunders, Philadelphia, pp 1401–1443
22. Markolf KL, Bargar WL, Shoemaker SC, Amstutz HC (1981) The role of joint load in knee stability. J Bone Joint Surg Am 63:570–585
23. Noyes FR, Barber-Westin SD, Hewett TE (2000) High tibial osteotomy and ligament reconstruction for varus angulated anterior cruciate ligament-deficient knees. Am J Sports Med 28:282–296
24. Hughston JC, Jacobson KE (1985) Chronic posterolateral rotatory instability of the knee. J Bone Joint Surg Am 67:351–359
25. Goradia VK, Van Allen J (2002) Chronic lateral knee instability treated with a high tibial osteotomy. Arthroscopy 18:807–811

26. Hetsroni I, Lyman S, Pearle AD, Marx RG (2013) The effect of lateral opening wedge distal femoral osteotomy on medial knee opening: clinical and biomechanical factors. Knee Surg Sports Traumatol Arthrosc. doi:10.1007/s00167-013-2405-3
27. Clatworthy M, Amendola A (1999) The anterior cruciate ligament and arthritis. Clin Sports Med 18:173–198
28. Naudie DD, Amendola A, Fowler PJ (2004) Opening wedge high tibial osteotomy for symptomatic hyperextension-varus thrust. Am J Sports Med 32:60–70
29. Ducat A, Sariali E, Lebel B, Mertl P, Hernigou P, Flecher X, Zayni R, Bonnin M, Jalil R, Amzallag J, Rosset P, Servien E, Gaudot F, Judet T, Catonné Y (2012) Posterior tibial slope changes after opening- and closing-wedge high tibial osteotomy: a comparative prospective multicenter study. Orthop Traumatol Surg Res 98(1):68–74
30. Noyes FR, Goebel SX, West J (2005) Opening wedge tibial osteotomy: the 3-triangle method to correct axial alignment and tibial slope. Am J Sports Med 33:378–387
31. Lerat JL, Moyen B, Garin C, Mandrino A, Besse JL, Brunet- Guedj E (1993) Anterior laxity and internal arthritis of the knee. Results of the reconstruction of the anterior cruciate ligament associated with tibial osteotomy. Rev Chir Orthop Reparatrice Appar Mot 79:365–374
32. Hohmann E, Bryant A, Imhoff AB (2006) The effect of closed wedge high tibial osteotomy on tibial slope: a radiographic study. Knee Surg Sports Traumatol Arthrosc 14:454–459
33. Giffin JR, Vogrin TM, Zantop T, Woo SL, Harner CD (2004) Effects of increasing tibial slope on the biomechanics of the knee. Am J Sports Med 32:376–382
34. Noyes FR, Barber-Westin SD (1996) Surgical restoration to treat chronic deficiency of the posterolateral complex and cruciate ligaments of the knee joint. Am J Sports Med 24:415–426
35. Aggarwal A, Panarella L, Amendola A (2005) Considerations for osteotomy in the ACL deficient knee. Sports Med Arthrosc 13:109–115
36. Dietrick T, Bugbee W (2005) Distal femoral osteotomy utilizing a lateral opening-wedge technique. Tech Knee Surg 4:186–192
37. Brown G, Amendola A (2000) Radiographic evaluation and preoperative planning for high tibial osteotomies. Oper Tech Sports Med 8:2–14
38. Savarese E, Bisicchia S, Romeo R, Amendola A (2011) Role of high tibial osteotomy in chronic injuries of posterior cruciate ligament and posterolateral corner. J Orthop Traumatol 12(1):1–17
39. LaPrade RF, Wentorf F (2002) Diagnosis and treatment of posterolateral knee injuries. Clin Orthop Relat Res 402:110–121
40. Dugdale TW, Noyes FR, Styer D (1992) Preoperative planning for high tibial osteotomy. The effect of lateral tibiofemoral separation and tibiofemoral length. Clin Orthop Relat Res 274:248–264
41. Rodner CM, Adams DJ, Diaz-Doran V, Tate JP, Santangelo SA, Mazzocca AD, Arciero RA (2006) Medial opening wedge tibial osteotomy and the sagittal plane: the effect of increasing tibial slope on tibiofemoral contact pressure. Am J Sports Med 34:1431–1441
42. Rossi R, Bonasia DE, Amendola A (2011) The role of high tibial osteotomy in the varus knee. J Am Acad Orthop Surg 19(10):593–596
43. Chou YC, Chen DC, Hsieh WA, Chen WF, Yen PS, Harnod T, Chiou TL, Chang YL, Su CF, Lin SZ, Chen SY (2008) Efficacy of anterior cervical fusion: comparison of titanium cages, polyetheretherketone (PEEK) cages and autogenous bone grafts. J Clin Neurosci 15:1240–1245
44. Getgood A, Collins B, Slynarski K, Kurowska E, Parker D, Engebretsen L, MacDonald PB, Litchfield R (2013) Short-term safety and efficacy of a novel high tibial osteotomy system: a case controlled study. Knee Surg Sports Traumatol Arthrosc 21(1):260–269
45. Fowler PJ, Kirkley A, Roe J (1994) Osteotomy of the proximal tibia in the treatment of chronic anterior cruciate ligament insufficiency. J Bone Joint Surg Br 76B(Suppl):26
46. Noyes FR, Dunworth LA, Andriacchi TP, Andrews M, Hewett TE (1996) Knee hyperextension gait abnormalities in unstable knees. Recognition and preoperative gait retraining. Am J Sports Med 24:35–45

47. Dejour H, Neyret P, Boileau P, Donell ST (1994) Anterior cruciate reconstruction combined with valgus tibial osteotomy. Clin Orthop Relat Res 299:220–228
48. Boss A, Stutz G, Oursin C, Gächter A (1995) Anterior cruciate ligament reconstruction combined with valgus tibial osteotomy (combined procedure). Knee Surg Sports Traumatol Arthrosc 3:187–191
49. Arthur A, LaPrade RF, Agel J (2007) Proximal tibial opening wedge osteotomy as the initial treatment for chronic posterolateral corner deficiency in the varus knee: a prospective clinical study. Am J Sports Med 35(11):1844–1850

Combined ACL and Peripheral Instability: The Eastern Experience

11

Ryosuke Kuroda, Takehiko Matsushita, Daisuke Araki, Yuichiro Nishizawa, Tomoyuki Matsumoto, and Masahiro Kurosaka

11.1 Introduction

Anterior cruciate ligament (ACL) reconstruction has become one of the more common procedures performed by orthopedic surgeons over the past 20 years. Successful long-term results are achieved in 75–95 % of these patients, but 8 % have unsatisfactory results due to recurrent instability and graft failure [1–3]. To prevent failure of ACL reconstruction, surgeons should understand ACL anatomy and surgical technique of anatomic ACL reconstruction. Also surgeons should understand that successful ACL reconstruction does not depend only on surgery itself but also on other factors, such as combined other soft tissue injuries, postoperative rehabilitation/training for returning to sports, and risk factors of reinjury and failure of graft incorporation. It has been reported that only 30–40 % of patients were rated as normal in International Knee Documentation Committee scores after single-bundle reconstruction and more than 60 % of patients may not make a full recovery to pre-injury levels [4]. In addition, it has been suggested that the single-bundle reconstruction did not fully restore normal knee kinematics by biomechanical studies [5, 6]. Anatomic studies have shown that native ACL is composed of two functional bundles, anteromedial (AM) and posterolateral (PL) bundles [7–9]. Therefore, there has been an increased interest in double-bundle ACL reconstruction, which replicates the two functional bundles, to more closely restore normal knee stability and kinematics [10–14]. In this chapter, we discussed about ACL instability and its treatment in the eastern experience. It has been reported that significant anterior subluxation of the tibia relative to femur at knee full extension was found in chronic ACL deficient-knees compared with the ACL intact-subjects [15, 16]. Moreover, chronic ACL deficiency causes anterior tibial subluxation, and anterior tibial subluxation was

R. Kuroda, MD, PhD (✉) • T. Matsushita, MD, PhD • D. Araki, MD, PhD
Y. Nishizawa, MD • T. Matsumoto, MD, PhD • M. Kurosaka, MD, PhD
Department of Orthopaedic Surgery, Kobe University Graduate School of Medicine,
7-5-2 Kusunoki-cho, Chuo-ku, Kobe 650-0017, Japan
e-mail: kurodar@med.kobe-u.ac.jp

R. Rossi, F. Margheritini (eds.), *Knee Ligament Injuries*,
DOI 10.1007/978-88-470-5513-1_11,

correlated positively with the duration of ACL deficiency and the extent of anterior instability [17]. To prevent failure of ACL reconstruction, biological integration of the grafted tendon is a crucial prerequisite for successful ACL reconstruction [18]. Theoretically, preservation of the biological and mechanical properties of the ACL remnant tissue may be able to restore proprioceptive function of the graft after ACL reconstruction [19]. ACL remnant has been demonstrated in experimental studies to have a role in improving revascularization, ligamentization, and reinnervation of the graft. Histological studies showed that the human ACL remnants contain a cellular capacity for healing potential [20–23]. In this chapter, we discuss about ACL instability and its treatment in the eastern experience in the following topics: anterior tibial subluxation in ACL-deficient knee, extra-articular reconstruction in ACL-deficient knee, remnant preservation surgery, and augmentation reconstruction.

11.2 Anterior Tibial Subluxation Before and After ACL Reconstruction

ACL-deficient knees had not only anterior instability but also anterior tibial subluxation to femur at full knee extension compared with ACL-intact knees [15, 16, 24]. Mishima et al. reported that anterior tibial subluxation in ACL-deficient knees was correlated positively with the time from initial injury and anterior instability (side-to-side difference) measured by KT-1000 [17]. It has been indicated that in the time since injury, ACL deficiency induced pathologic changes of other soft tissues over time and led to anterior tibial subluxation. In the anterior instability, patients with significant instability had low resistance to anterior tibial translation, and it induced secondary changes such as shortening of the posterior cruciate ligament (PCL) and/or posterior capsule, which led to anterior tibial subluxation.

Moreover, Fukuta et al. reported anterior tibial subluxation was significantly larger in patients with a history of reinjury, injury to the medial and lateral meniscus, and the presence of gross pivot shift [25].

On the other hand, it has been reported that even in patients with clinically successful ACL reconstruction, anterior tibial subluxation could not be restored with a posteriorly directed force on the tibia and there was residual fixed anterior tibial subluxation after ACL reconstruction [15, 16, 26]. It was suggested that the violated synovial sheath of the intact PCL may cause a scarring response and a subsequent contracture of PCL, which could explain the fixed anterior subluxation after ACL reconstruction. A similar phenomenon, characterized by morphological changes in ACL [27] and an irreducible posterior subluxation [28], has been reported in knees with an intact ACL and a chronically deficient PCL.

Furthermore, Almekinders et al. also reported that osteoarthritic changes following untreated ACL-deficient knees were associated with uncorrectable anterior tibial subluxation along with a decrease in instability. The irreducible tibial anterior subluxation could explain why osteoarthritic changes still may develop in stable, reconstructed knees in spite of the improved stability [26].

In our study, ACL-deficient knees with more than 6 months after initial injury had significantly larger anterior tibial subluxation, and it was difficult to reduce anterior tibial subluxation after ACL reconstruction in chronic ACL-deficient knees with large tibial subluxation.

11.3 The Combined Intra- and Extra-articular Reconstruction in the Eastern Experience

Yamaguchi et al. [29] reported the combined intra- and extra-articular ACL reconstruction with iliotibial tract (45 patients). Surgical procedure consisted of intra- and extra-articular reconstruction with ITT. A 25-cm longitudinal incision that dissected the subcutaneous tissue was made on the lateral aspect of the thigh. A 22-cm strip of the ITT graft was harvested, leaving the tibial insertion (Gerdy's tubercle) attached. A femoral tunnel was drilled in an outside-in fashion. The intra-articular outlet was the superomedial corner of the lateral femoral condyle, just anterior to the joint capsule. A separate medial parapatellar incision was made. A tibial tunnel was drilled under direct vision from medial to tibial tuberosity to the anterior half of the ACL stump. The graft was passed deep to the fibular collateral ligament and through the femoral and tibial tunnels. With the knee at 90° of flexion and the foot externally rotated, the graft was pulled taut and sutured to the fibular collateral ligament and the periosteum of lateral femoral condyle. Then, with the knee at 30° flexion and the foot kept externally rotated, the graft was sutured to the periosteum around the outlet of the tibial tunnel. They also reported the clinical results of 24-year follow-up and that 17 (71 %) patients had moderate or severe degenerative changes on radiographs although about 50 % of the patients participated in regular sports activities and no patient required regular clinical intervention [29]. In this clinical study, it has been still unknown that the combined intra- and extra-articular ACL reconstruction could restore normal knee kinematics or not (Fig. 11.1).

11.4 Remnant Preservation Surgery in the Eastern Experience

Remnant preserved anterior cruciate ligament (ACL) reconstruction, which is designed to preserve the ACL remnant, has become increasingly popular over the last decade [19, 30–36]. Since Schultz et al. reported the first detailed description of mechanoreceptors in the ACL [37], the ACL remnant has been recognized in terms of its proprioceptive functions and its vascularity, which may induce more rapid vascularization from the ACL remnant to the grafts [27, 38, 39]. Theoretically, there is a strong possibility that preservation of the ACL remnant tissue may be able to restore proprioceptive function of the graft after ACL reconstruction. Preservation of the ACL remnant tissue may also enhance the revascularization and cellular proliferation of the graft after ACL reconstruction since the ACL remnant tissue has good subsynovial and intrafascicular vascularity [40]. Based on these concepts,

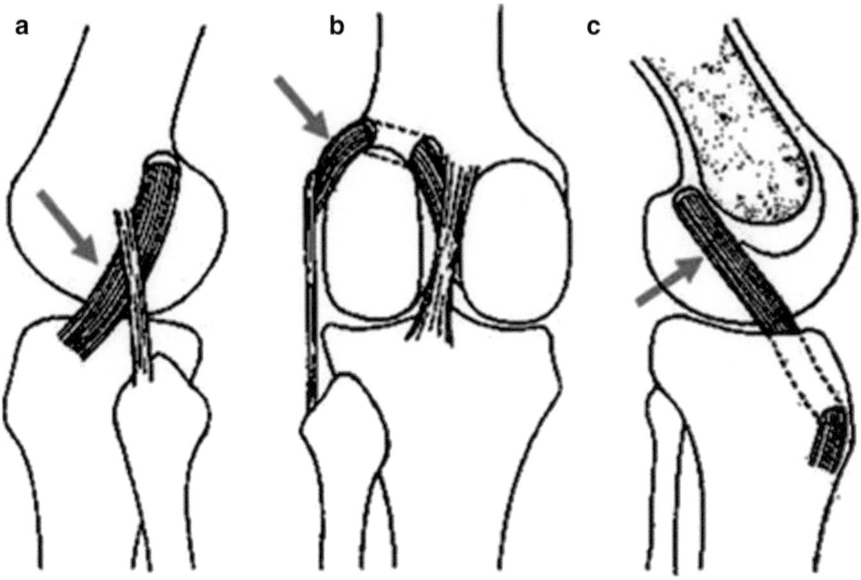

Fig. 11.1 The combined intra- and extra-articular ACL reconstruction reported by Yamaguchi et al. Lateral (**a**), posterior (**b**), and intercondylar (**c**) views of their ACL reconstruction technique. Combined intra- and extra-articular reconstruction with iliotibial tract was performed. (→): The ACL graft.

several investigators have developed single-bundle ACL reconstruction techniques with preservation of the ACL remnant tissue [31, 32, 34, 35]. Recently, Ahn et al. introduced a remnant preserving technique for double-bundle ACL reconstruction, in which two femoral tunnels and one tibial tunnel are created [33]. Subsequently, Ochi et al. described a double-bundle ACL reconstruction with remnant preserving technique using a hamstring autograft [30]. They utilize the far anteromedial portal to create the femoral tunnels and the central anteromedial portal to make a longitudinal slit in the ACL remnant to allow visualization of the tips of the guide pins during anatomic creation of the tibial tunnels within the native ACL tibial footprint. Yasuda et al. reported the clinical outcomes of the anatomic double-bundle ACL reconstruction with ligament remnant tissue preservation by the use of the transtibial technique [19]. They concluded that the results of this technique were comparable to their previously reported results of anatomic double-bundle reconstruction without remnant tissue preservation. The most important factor of this technique is the evaluation of ACL remnant tissue. To accurately evaluate the morphology of the remnants, arthroscopic examination should be performed at various knee flexion angles to consider the different tension patterns of the two bundles (anteromedial bundle (AMB) and posterolateral bundle (PLB)). The status of the PLB femoral insertion can be evaluated with the knee in a figure-of-4 position for good visualization of the femoral attachment. Most of the ACL remnants do not play a role for biomechanical function. In addition, no long-term studies have shown clinical evidence regarding the utility of ACL remnant tissue preservation, and this technique demands a high level of surgical skills. Anatomic placement of femoral and tibial tunnels should be the basis of ACL reconstruction in order to obtain optimal clinical and biomechanical results.

11.5 Augmentation Reconstruction in the Eastern Experience

On the other hand, some of the ACL remnants are identified as an isolated AMB or PLB tear. To identify these types of rupture pattern, careful arthroscopic inspection is the key. First, the locations of the femoral and tibial attachment are evaluated carefully. Second, the directions of the remaining fibers are assessed. Both of these procedures are performed at 90° of knee flexion. If the AMB is intact, the remnant bundle, which connects the AMB insertion site between the femur and the tibia, is tightened with probing at this angle. The remnant bundles are also subsequently evaluated in a figure-of-4 position. When the PLB is intact, the tightened remnant bundle is observed. Nakamae et al. evaluated the biomechanical function of ACL remnants in anterior-posterior and rotational knee stability in patients with a complete ACL injury [41]. They classified the ACL remnants into five morphological patterns by arthroscopic inspection. In these five groups, they demonstrated that patients with partial AMB or PLB rupture had a significantly lesser amount of anterior-posterior translation by KT-2000 measurement. Our previous report by Araki et al. also evaluated the partial rupture of AMB or PLB using the electromagnetic measurement system (EMS) [42]. The quantitative assessments of knees with partial ACL ruptures during the Lachman and the pivot shift tests using the EMS showed less laxity than knees with complete ACL tears, whereas their laxity was greater than the contralateral knees with intact ACLs. Therefore, ACL remnants that can be confirmed by careful inspection as almost completely preserving the AMB or PLB should be considered as partial ACL tears. It is suggested that these ACL remnants contribute to the knee joint stability seen in our study. Based on these findings, ACL augmentation technique, which reproduces selective AMB or PLB reconstruction, has been performed and resulted in the good clinical score. Ochi et al. examined the 2-year follow-up clinical results of 45 patients who had undergone ACL augmentation procedure using an autogenous semitendinosus tendon [43]. When the ACL remnant was regarded as a PLB, only the AMB was reconstructed. In contrast, when the ACL remnant was regarded as an AMB, only the PLB was reconstructed. This procedure showed improved postoperative joint stability, joint position sense, and Lysholm scores. They concluded that this procedure can be a treatment option for patients whose ACL remnants are left in certain conditions. A recent study by Ohsawa et al. also evaluated the clinical results and morphology of the preserved bundle remnants by second-look arthroscopy postoperatively 1 year after selective AMB or PLB ACL reconstruction [44]. They reported that the preserved ACL remnants possessed acceptable morphology and the functions of anterior-posterior and rotational stability after surgery. To successfully perform this technique, it is important to first identify the partial ACL tear, which is almost completely preserved as the AMB or PLB. The augmentation reconstruction technique can be performed less invasively by preservation of these bundles. In addition, the biomechanical function and biological healings are enhanced by preservation of these residual bundles. Therefore, although this technique is also technically demanding, this procedure can be a treatment option for patients whose ACL remnants are left in certain conditions.

11.6 Summary

We reviewed ACL instability and its treatment in the eastern experience. Chronic ACL-deficient knees had significantly larger anterior tibial subluxation, and it was difficult to reduce anterior tibial subluxation after ACL reconstruction in chronic ACL-deficient knees and large tibial subluxation cases. Regarding the combined intra- and extra-articular reconstruction, it is still unknown whether these surgical procedures could restore normal knee kinematics or not in the literature, and we could not find any advantages so far. From the previous clinical studies in Japan, anatomic reconstruction is crucial to restore normal knee kinematics. In addition, the biomechanical function and biological healings are enhanced by preservation of ACL remnant. Therefore, we believe that although this procedure is technically demanding, anatomic double-bundle ACL reconstruction with ACL remnant preservation has been a better treatment option to restore normal knee kinematics.

References

1. Corsetti JR, Jackson DW (1996) Failure of anterior cruciate ligament reconstruction: the biologic basis. Clin Orthop Relat Res 325:42–49
2. Getelman MH, Friedman MJ (1999) Revision anterior cruciate ligament reconstruction surgery. J Am Acad Orthop Surg 7(3):189–198
3. Jaureguito JW, Paulos LE (1996) Why grafts fail. Clin Orthop Relat Res 325:25–41
4. Biau DJ, Tournoux C, Katsahian S, Schranz P, Nizard R (2007) ACL reconstruction: a meta-analysis of functional scores. Clin Orthop Relat Res 458:180–187
5. Georgoulis AD, Papadonikolakis A, Papageorgiou CD, Mitsou A, Stergiou N (2003) Three-dimensional tibiofemoral kinematics of the anterior cruciate ligament-deficient and reconstructed knee during walking. Am J Sports Med 31(1):75–79
6. Woo SL, Kanamori A, Zeminski J, Yagi M, Papageorgiou C, Fu FH (2002) The effectiveness of reconstruction of the anterior cruciate ligament with hamstrings and patellar tendon. A cadaveric study comparing anterior tibial and rotational loads. J Bone Joint Surg Am 84-A(6):907–914
7. Girgis FG, Marshall JL, Monajem A (1975) The cruciate ligaments of the knee joint. Anatomical, functional and experimental analysis. Clin Orthop Relat Res (106):216–231
8. Arnoczky SP (1983) Anatomy of the anterior cruciate ligament. Clin Orthop Relat Res 172:19–25
9. Amis AA, Dawkins GP (1991) Functional anatomy of the anterior cruciate ligament. Fibre bundle actions related to ligament replacements and injuries. J Bone Joint Surg Br 73(2): 260–267
10. Mae T, Shino K, Miyama T et al (2001) Single- versus two-femoral socket anterior cruciate ligament reconstruction technique: biomechanical analysis using a robotic simulator. Arthroscopy 17(7):708–716

11. Musahl V, Voos JE, O'Loughlin PF et al (2010) Comparing stability of different single- and double-bundle anterior cruciate ligament reconstruction techniques: a cadaveric study using navigation. Arthroscopy 26(9 Suppl):S41–S48
12. Yagi M, Wong EK, Kanamori A, Debski RE, Fu FH, Woo SL (2002) Biomechanical analysis of an anatomic anterior cruciate ligament reconstruction. Am J Sports Med 30(5):660–666
13. Kuroda R, Matsushita T (2011) Anatomic double-bundle anterior crucial ligament reconstruction with G-ST. Curr Rev Musculoskelet Med 4(2):57–64
14. Fujita N, Kuroda R, Matsumoto T et al (2011) Comparison of the clinical outcome of double-bundle, anteromedial single-bundle, and posterolateral single-bundle anterior cruciate ligament reconstruction using hamstring tendon graft with minimum 2-year follow-up. Arthroscopy 27(7):906–913
15. Almekinders LC, Chiavetta JB (2001) Tibial subluxation in anterior cruciate ligament-deficient knees: implications for tibial tunnel placement. Arthroscopy 17(9):960–962
16. Almekinders LC, de Castro D (2001) Fixed tibial subluxation after successful anterior cruciate ligament reconstruction. Am J Sports Med 29(3):280–283
17. Mishima S, Takahashi S, Kondo S, Ishiguro N (2005) Anterior tibial subluxation in anterior cruciate ligament-deficient knees: quantification using magnetic resonance imaging. Arthroscopy 21(10):1193–1196
18. Locherbach C, Zayni R, Chambat P, Sonnery-Cottet B (2010) Biologically enhanced ACL reconstruction. Orthop Traumatol Surg Res 96(7):810–815
19. Yasuda K, Kondo E, Kitamura N, Kawaguchi Y, Kai S, Tanabe Y (2012) A pilot study of anatomic double-bundle anterior cruciate ligament reconstruction with ligament remnant tissue preservation. Arthroscopy 28(3):343–353
20. Matsumoto T, Ingham SM, Mifune Y et al (2012) Isolation and characterization of human anterior cruciate ligament-derived vascular stem cells. Stem Cells Dev 21(6):859–872
21. Matsumoto T, Kubo S, Sasaki K et al (2012) Acceleration of tendon-bone healing of anterior cruciate ligament graft using autologous ruptured tissue. Am J Sports Med 40(6): 1296–1302
22. Mifune Y, Matsumoto T, Ota S et al (2012) Therapeutic potential of anterior cruciate ligament-derived stem cells for anterior cruciate ligament reconstruction. Cell Transplant 21(8):1651–1665
23. Mifune Y, Matsumoto T, Takayama K et al (2013) Tendon graft revitalization using adult anterior cruciate ligament (ACL)-derived CD34+ cell sheets for ACL reconstruction. Biomaterials 34(22):5476–5487
24. Vahey TN, Hunt JE, Shelbourne KD (1993) Anterior translocation of the tibia at MR imaging: a secondary sign of anterior cruciate ligament tear. Radiology 187(3):817–819
25. Fukuta H, Takahashi S, Hasegawa Y, Ida K, Iwata H (2000) Passive terminal extension causes anterior tibial translation in some anterior cruciate ligament-deficient knees. J Orthop Sci 5(3):192–197
26. Almekinders LC, Pandarinath R, Rahusen FT (2004) Knee stability following anterior cruciate ligament rupture and surgery. The contribution of irreducible tibial subluxation. J Bone Joint Surg Am 86-A(5):983–987
27. Ochi M, Murao T, Sumen Y, Kobayashi K, Adachi N (1999) Isolated posterior cruciate ligament insufficiency induces morphological changes of anterior cruciate ligament collagen fibrils. Arthroscopy 15(3):292–296
28. Strobel MJ, Weiler A, Schulz MS, Russe K, Eichhorn HJ (2002) Fixed posterior subluxation in posterior cruciate ligament-deficient knees: diagnosis and treatment of a new clinical sign. Am J Sports Med 30(1):32–38
29. Yamaguchi S, Sasho T, Tsuchiya A, Wada Y, Moriya H (2006) Long term results of anterior cruciate ligament reconstruction with iliotibial tract: 6-, 13-, and 24-year longitudinal follow-up. Knee Surg Sports Traumatol Arthrosc 14(11):1094–1100
30. Ochi M, Abouheif MM, Kongcharoensombat W, Nakamae A, Adachi N, Deie M (2011) Double bundle arthroscopic Anterior Cruciate Ligament reconstruction with remnant preserving technique using a hamstring autograft. Sports Med Arthrosc Rehabil Ther Technol 3:30

31. Adachi N, Ochi M, Uchio Y, Sumen Y (2000) Anterior cruciate ligament augmentation under arthroscopy. A minimum 2-year follow-up in 40 patients. Arch Orthop Trauma Surg 120(3–4):128–133
32. Ochi M, Adachi N, Deie M, Kanaya A (2006) Anterior cruciate ligament augmentation procedure with a 1-incision technique: anteromedial bundle or posterolateral bundle reconstruction. Arthroscopy 22(4):463.e1–463.e5
33. Ahn JH, Lee YS, Ha HC (2009) Anterior cruciate ligament reconstruction with preservation of remnant bundle using hamstring autograft: technical note. Arch Orthop Trauma Surg 129(8):1011–1015
34. Lee BI, Kwon SW, Kim JB, Choi HS, Min KD (2008) Comparison of clinical results according to amount of preserved remnant in arthroscopic anterior cruciate ligament reconstruction using quadrupled hamstring graft. Arthroscopy 24(5):560–568
35. Lee BI, Min KD, Choi HS, Kim JB, Kim ST (2006) Arthroscopic anterior cruciate ligament reconstruction with the tibial-remnant preserving technique using a hamstring graft. Arthroscopy 22(3):340.e1–340.e7
36. Yoon KH, Bae DK, Cho SM, Park SY, Lee JH (2009) Standard anterior cruciate ligament reconstruction versus isolated single-bundle augmentation with hamstring autograft. Arthroscopy 25(11):1265–1274
37. Schultz RA, Miller DC, Kerr CS, Micheli L (1984) Mechanoreceptors in human cruciate ligaments. A histological study. J Bone Joint Surg Am 66(7):1072–1076
38. Adachi N, Ochi M, Uchino Y, Iwasa J, Ryoke K, Kuriwaka M (2002) Contribution of mechanoreceptors in the anterior cruciate ligament to the joint position sense knee. Acta Orthop Scand 73:330–334
39. Mifune Y, Ota S, Takayama K et al (2013) Therapeutic advantage in selective ligament augmentation for partial tears of the anterior cruciate ligament: results in an animal model. Am J Sports Med 41(2):365–373
40. Dhillon MS, Bali K, Vasistha RK (2010) Immunohistological evaluation of proprioceptive potential of the residual stump of injured anterior cruciate ligaments (ACL). Int Orthop 34(5):737–741
41. Nakamae A, Ochi M, Deie M et al (2010) Biomechanical function of anterior cruciate ligament remnants: how long do they contribute to knee stability after injury in patients with complete tears? Arthroscopy 26(12):1577–1585
42. Araki D, Kuroda R, Matsushita T et al (2013) Biomechanical analysis of the knee with partial anterior cruciate ligament disruption: quantitative evaluation using an electromagnetic measurement system. Arthroscopy 29(6):1053–1062
43. Ochi M, Adachi N, Uchio Y et al (2009) A minimum 2-year follow-up after selective anteromedial or posterolateral bundle anterior cruciate ligament reconstruction. Arthroscopy 25(2):117–122
44. Ohsawa T, Kimura M, Kobayashi Y, Hagiwara K, Yorifuji H, Takagishi K (2012) Arthroscopic evaluation of preserved ligament remnant after selective anteromedial or posterolateral bundle anterior cruciate ligament reconstruction. Arthroscopy 28(6):807–817

Combined ACL and Peripheral Instability: The Western Experience

12

Stefano Zaffagnini, Alberto Grassi, Tommaso Roberti di Sarsina, Tommaso Bonanzinga, Giulio Maria Marcheggiani Muccioli, and Maurilio Marcacci

12.1 Introduction

In this chapter, we will analyze our experience concerning ACL lesion with an associated peripheral instability, as peripheral structures are getting more and more attention studying primary ACL reconstruction failure causes. We know that the combined damage of the ACL and the posterolateral structures of the knee has been associated to chronic anterior cruciate ligament laxity, in particular rotational laxity associated with a severe pivot shift test (PST) [1, 2]. The Segond fracture that results from avulsion of the iliotibial band (ITB) or the "anterior oblique band" of the lateral collateral ligament (LCL) is often encountered along with ACL tears and considered possible evidence of damage of these structures [3]. It is common to find also "bone bruising" upon observing magnetic resonance images as a result of the lateral tibial subluxation due to gross instability after ACL and lateral structure damage [4, 5]. As Dodds and Amis have recently published, these posterolateral structures may not have been yet directly identified, but probably act as secondary restraints to the PST, supplementing the primary restraint role of the ACL in anteroposterior laxity, with emphasis on rotatory laxity and internal rotation [6]. The persistence of this rotatory laxity has been reported even after cases of uneventful ACL reconstruction, suggesting that a single-bundle intra-articular reconstruction could not be sufficient to completely restore rotational knee stability in certain patients [7]. These are some of the concerns that led professor Marcacci to the development of his single-bundle over-the-top ACL reconstruction plus lateral plasty that we adopted in our institute since 1993. This technique makes allowance for three considerations: the previously mentioned

S. Zaffagnini (✉) • A. Grassi • T.R. di Sarsina • T. Bonanzinga
G.M.M. Muccioli • M. Marcacci
Clinica Ortopedica e Traumatologica II, Laboratorio di Biomeccanica ed Innovazione Tecnologica, Istituto Ortopedico Rizzoli, Via di Barbiano, 1/10, Bologna 40136, Italy
e-mail: stefano.zaffagnini@biomec.ior.it; alberto.grassi@ior.it; tommaso.robertidisarsina@hotmail.com; tommaso.bonanzinga@ior.it; marcheggianimuccioli@me.com; m.marcacci@biomec.ior.it

R. Rossi, F. Margheritini (eds.), *Knee Ligament Injuries*,
DOI 10.1007/978-88-470-5513-1_12, © Springer Verlag Italia 2014

evidence of the *additional structures being damaged* in ACL tears favors that there are *additional structures required to be addressed* in ACL reconstruction, the fact that posterolateral structures are crucial in controlling internal tibial rotation, and that the lateral extra-articular plasty is far from the center of the knee rotation and provides a greater lever arm for controlling PST and internal rotation than the intra-articular reconstruction [8]. The rationale behind extra-articular plasty is therefore to create a restraint in internal tibial rotation. Authors who favor the supplementary extra-articular plasty to standard ACL reconstruction report the reduction of the PST and lateral tibial translation [9]; however, the introduction of evidence-based inclusion criteria for any similar technique as a primary or a revision option is difficult and remains sporadical and empirically based [10].

12.2 ACL Reconstruction + Lateral Plasty: Surgical Technique

12.2.1 Arthroscopic Setting

The patient is positioned supine on the operating table, with a pneumatic tourniquet as high as possible around the proximal part of the thigh. A support is placed laterally at the upper level of the knee to stress the joint during arthroscopic evaluation. Usually a medial suprapatellar portal is used for the water inflow, as well as an anterolateral viewing portal and an anteromedial working portal. Meniscectomies or chondroplasty is performed where necessary. When ACL lesion is confirmed, the tibial insertion area and the intercondylar notch are prepared. The tibial insertion is preserved, while the notch is cleared from soft tissues without making a real "notchplasty."

12.2.2 Graft Harvesting

The patient's leg is positioned in a figure 4 position; the pes anserinus is located by following the hamstring tendons distally to their attachment on the anteromedial tibia. A 3 cm transverse incision is made over the pes anserinus (2 cm distal and 1 cm medial to the tibial tubercle). Subcutaneous tissue is then dissected, and the fascia is incised parallel to the orientation of the pes tendons (Fig. 12.1). The sartorius tendon is retracted superiorly, and the gracilis and semitendinosus tendons are bluntly dissected from the surrounding soft tissue. Both tendons are harvested using a blunt tendon stripper (Acufex, Microsurgical, Mansfield, MA) while maintaining firm tension on the tendon distally and with the knee in more than 90° flexion to facilitate the detachment of the tendon. In order to obtain the maximum length possible of the graft, which is usually about 20 cm long, extra care should be taken. The harvested tendons are then sutured together using three nonabsorbable Flexidene no. 2 stitches (Laboratory Bruneau, Boulogne Billancourt, France), and the sutures are tightened, with emphasis at the free proximal tendon ends. The tibial insertion of both tendons is preserved to maintain their neurovascular supply.

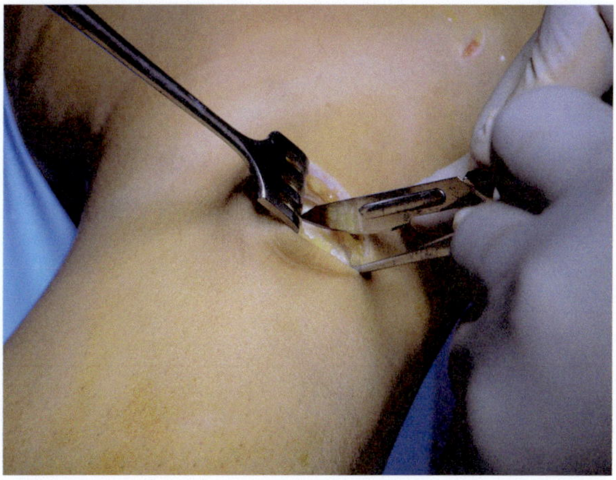

Fig. 12.1 Incision of the fascia parallel to the orientation of the pes anserinus tendons

12.2.3 Tibial Tunnel

Under arthroscopic visualization, a guide pin is inserted on the medial aspect of the tibia through the graft harvesting incision, directed to the medial posterior part of the ACL tibial insertion. The guide pin is usually reamed with a diameter of 8–9 mm. Then, a looped wire passer is inserted from the tibial tunnel into the notch and is brought out from the anteromedial portal with a forceps.

12.2.4 Over-the-Top Position

The knee is then positioned at 90° flexion with the foot externally rotated, and a longitudinal incision 3–5 cm long is made directly above the lateral femoral epicondyle. The posterior third of the iliotibial band is divided and is retracted anteriorly. In order to reach the lateral intermuscular septum, which separates the vastus lateralis muscle (above) from the lateral head of the gastrocnemius muscle (below), we dissect the lateral aspect of the thigh. When the lateral intermuscular septum has been clearly identified, it is possible to reach the posterior aspect of the joint capsule by passing over this structure. If this is not possible, the septum can be divided. By palpating the posterior tubercle of the lateral femoral condyle with a finger, it is possible to determine the correct placement of the "over-the-top" position and to protect the posterior structures during the next step. A curved Kelly clamp is inserted into the anteromedial portal directed to the notch, and its tip is placed as far proximally possible against the posterior part of the capsule. After palpating the tip of the clamp from the lateral side of the femur just posterior to the intermuscular septum, it is pushed through the thin posterior layer of the knee capsule, reaching the posterior space previously prepared. A suture loop is then placed into the tip of the clamp, pulled anteriorly through the anteromedial portal, and placed into the wire loop previously inserted in the portal. Pulling the wire from the tibial side brings the

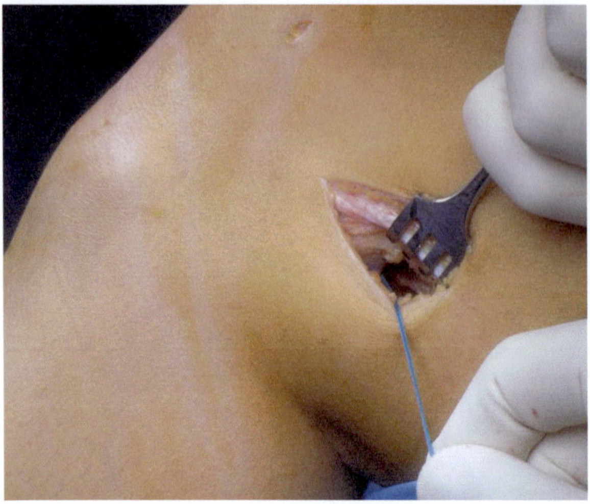

Fig. 12.2 The suture loop is pulled from the femoral incision to pass the graft through the knee joint

suture loop at the bottom of the tibial tunnel and out from the tibial incision. At the end of this step, the suture crosses the tibial tunnel and the knee joint exiting from the lateral incision (Fig. 12.2).

12.2.5 Graft Placement and Fixation

The free end of the graft is then tied to the passing suture, which is pulled through the knee joint retrieving the graft from the lateral incision using a small osteotome (Fig. 12.3). A groove is made in the lateral aspect of the femur just proximally to the start of the lateral condyle, allowing the anteriorization of the grafts and the achievement of a more isometric position. Once the graft is placed in the correct position, it is tensioned and the knee cycled through a full range of motion to check its stability. Then, the graft can be secured to the lateral femoral cortex into the groove with two metal staples (Fig. 12.4), while maintaining the knee at about 90° of flexion and the foot externally rotated. It is possible to check if the graft is long enough to perform lateral plasty, by putting it under tension directed to the anterolateral aspect of the tibia. If the graft is of the required length, a 1–2 cm skin and fascia incision is performed just below the GT (Fig. 12.5). Then, a small Kelly clamp is passed under the fascia from this incision to the lateral femoral condyle, where the sutures at the end of the graft are placed in the tip of the clamp and pulled down, emerging from the GT incision. After graft tensioning and after checking the isometry of the lateral tenodesis, another metallic staple is then used to fix the graft below GT to the lateral aspect of the tibia. An intra-articular drain is inserted through the superomedial portal, and another drain is inserted in the medial and lateral wounds. The iliotibial tract defect is closed, taking care to prevent lateral tilt and patellar compression, while the medial fascia over the pes anserinus is not closed

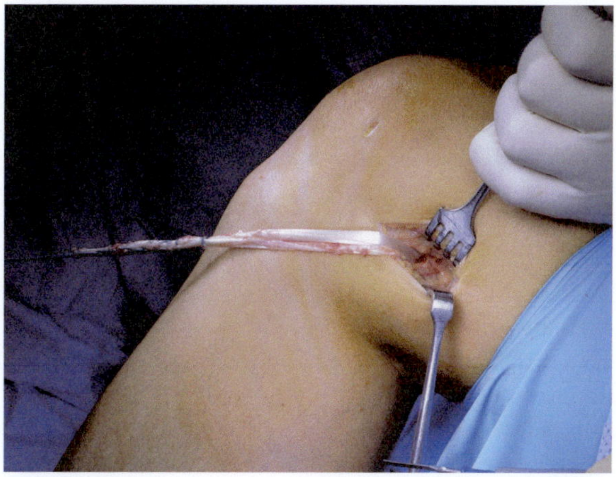

Fig. 12.3 After the graft exits from the lateral incision, its length is checked before proceeding with the lateral plasty

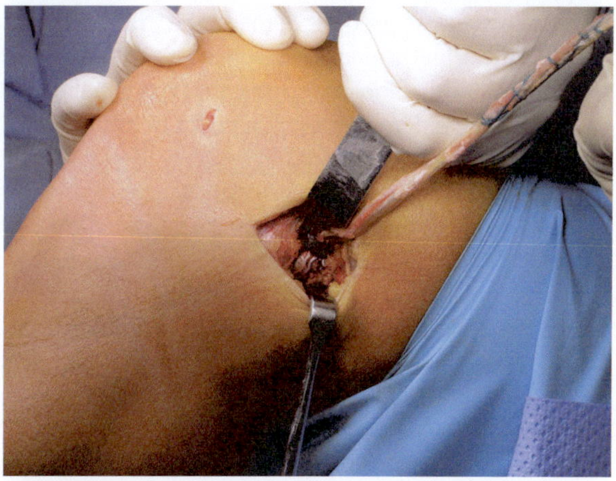

Fig. 12.4 The graft is fixed to the lateral femoral cortex with two staples, maintaining the knee at about 90° of flexion and the foot externally rotated

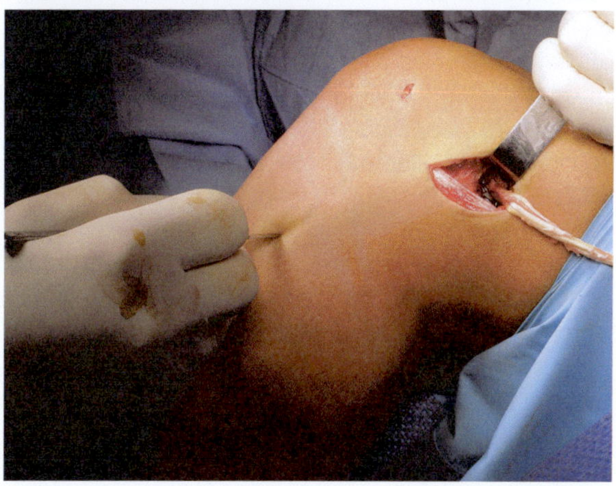

Fig. 12.5 After checking the correct length of the graft, a 1–2 cm incision is made just below the Gerdy tubercle to perform the lateral plasty

12.3 Pearls and Pitfalls

The main feature for the success of this technique is the adequate length of the graft; therefore, all events that could cause a short graft harvesting or graft rupture should be carefully avoided. A meticulous dissection of both gracilis and semitendinosus tendons from their fascial attachments is mandatory in order to prevent early cutting of the tendons when advancing the tendon stripper. If this event happens and one of the two tendons is shorter, the graft could be sutured in any case, and the reconstruction should be performed according to the described technique. In most of the cases, the intra-articular graft will be formed by two strands, while the lateral plasty will be inevitably formed by a biomechanically weaker single strand. In order to gain an additional 1 or 2 cm in length, the distal attachment of the semitendinosus to the adjacent gracilis tendon could be dissected. Another potential danger of the graft's integrity could be the sharpness of the edges of the tibial tunnel hole, and as tension is applied to the graft when passing through the tibial tunnel, it could produce a cutting mechanism that could damage the graft. Therefore, before passing the graft through the tibial tunnel, the edges of the osseous tunnel should be accurately smoothened with a motorized shaver. Detachment of the distal insertion of the tendons from the anteromedial tibia could be caused by excessive graft tensioning as well; therefore, the graft should be correctly tensioned with a progressive increase of the force avoiding rough stretches. In case of detachment of the distal insertion of the tendons, both the strands of the distal end of the graft could be sutured together, and the graft should be retrieved downwards through the tibial tunnel and fixed with an interference screw or metallic staple. At this point, the possibility to perform the lateral tenodesis depends on the remaining length of the graft. Additionally, the fixation of the graft with metallic staples, especially at the lateral femoral cortex, could be a source of graft damage, as the barb of the staple coupled with high tension applied to the graft could produce a guillotine effect. In order to avoid this drawback, the staples should be firmly fixed to the bone cortex, without driving them too deeply. On the other hand, a not firm fixation will lead to loss of proper graft tension and almost certain failure of the reconstruction. In case of graft rupture that does not allow the lateral tenodesis, the ACL reconstruction could be performed by maintaining only the intra-articular part, with all the limitations derived from a single-bundle nonanatomic technique.

Correct graft placement, both for the intra- and the extra-articular part, is mandatory in order to obtain good outcomes and avoid dangerous complications. Positioning the tibial tunnel to the posteromedial part of ACL tibial insertion, coupled with the use of the over-the-top position, guarantees the correct location of the graft, which is posteriorly enough to avoid impingement. Nevertheless, in chronic cases, big osteophytes, especially on the medial edge of the lateral condyle, could obstruct the intercondylar notch; therefore, a true notchplasty should be performed to avoid graft impingement. Any soft tissue in the posterior part of the roof that can obstruct the "over-the-top" position must be carefully removed as well. The incorrect placement of the extra-articular tenodesis could produce excessive tension on the graft along the range of motion, causing pain and joint stiffness. This could be avoided by fixing the graft in the isometric position. Creating a small groove in the lateral aspect of the femur allows the graft to move anteriorly, while the repeated cycling allows the construct to find its optimal placement for the distal fixation and to check the graft tension along the complete range of motion.

A special mention goes to a more dangerous and harmful complication related to this technique, which is the injury of the popliteal artery when approaching to the over-the-top position. Although this is a rare event, it should be considered as a vascular emergency and its treatment is beyond the scope of this chapter. But this risk is almost inconsistent, if all the steps are scrupulously followed.

12.4 Results

Marcacci et al. reported the long-term results of their nonanatomic over-the-top ACL reconstruction combined with lateral tenodesis using hamstring graft [11]. The authors recommended the technique for primary ACL reconstruction since they recorded that 90 % of the 54 consecutive cases scored "good" or "excellent" results in IKDC after an average of 11 years. Bignozzi et al. evaluated the results of the latter technique with computer-assisted navigation and found that the addition of an extra-articular procedure to the single-bundle ACL reconstruction successfully controlled coupled tibial translation during the Lachman test and reduced anteroposterior laxity at 90° of flexion [12]. Buda et al. utilized the same nonanatomic over-the-top technique using allograft tendons for multiple-revision ACL reconstruction, reporting "good" or "excellent" results in 83 % of patients and 92 % with "normal" to "nearly normal" PST [13]. Also, Trojani et al. reported the results of ACL revision with additional lateral plasty, although using different grafts, showing better results in terms of stability and failure rate compared to isolated intra-articular reconstruction [14]. Most of these authors agree that the critical point for the success of the extra-articular plasty is the point of femoral fixation [6, 8]. This has been defined to be located slightly posteriorly and proximally to the femoral insertion of the LCL [15]. Some authors have introduced navigation systems that help the surgeon to study the correct graft placement and kinematics and compare the results with the native contralateral ACL [16]. Colombet published a technique where he uses navigation in order to facilitate the identification of this femoral insertion point [17]. A reasonable argument in favor of supplementary extra-articular plasty is that it provides additional protection on the intra-articular reconstruction, especially in the early rehabilitation period. Even though the in vitro study of the extra-articular plasty showed that it decreases up to 43 % the forces upon the primary intra-articular construct [18], the direct clinical value of the addition of extra-articular plasty is yet to be proved [6]. The few available studies that compare the two options produce contradicting results. Earlier reports showed no clear differences between intra-articular reconstruction and the addition of extra-articular plasty and that there is no benefit from the supplementary procedure [19–21]. On the other hand, some authors recorded benefits from the addition of extra-articular plasty, such as better PST control [22], reduced tibial internal rotation, and better constraint of lateral tibial displacement [9, 10, 23, 24]. Monaco and Ferretti et al. recorded that the addition of extra-articular plasty significantly reduced internal tibial rotation at 30° of flexion when compared to single- or double-bundle ACL reconstruction [25]. Zaffagnini et al. compared single-bundle ACL reconstruction plus extra-articular plasty with patellar tendon and four-strand hamstring and found superior results for the extra-articular plasty group, in terms of subjective clinical findings and time to return to sports activities [24]. More recently, the same group compared double-bundle ACL reconstruction versus single-bundle ACL reconstruction with extra-articular plasty and recorded that the latter resulted in better control of static knee laxity, reduced mediolateral instability in early flexion, and reduced rotatory instability at 90° of flexion [9].

The technique presented is a highly reproducible procedure in our hands, with a high percentage of satisfactory results, and eliminates the risk of surgical error that may be associated with placement of the femoral tunnel, and it uses only 3 titanium staples for graft fixation, which results in a reduction of surgical costs. In conclusion, we found that a combination of single-bundle ACL reconstruction with hamstrings plus extra-articular augmentation is capable of maintaining good stability at more than 10 years' follow-up [11].

References

1. Bull AMJ, Amis AA (1998) The pivot-shift phenomenon: a clinical and biomechanical perspective. Knee 5(5):141–158
2. Norwood LA Jr, Andrews JR, Meisterling RC et al (1979) Acute anterolateral rotatory instability of the knee. J Bone Joint Surg Am 61(5):704–709
3. Campos JC, Chung CB, Lektrakul N et al (2001) Pathogenesis of the Segond fracture: anatomic and MR imaging evidence of an iliotibial tract or anterior oblique band avulsion. Radiology 219(2):381–386
4. Tashiro Y, Okazaki K, Miura H et al (2009) Quantitative assessment of rotatory instability after anterior cruciate ligament reconstruction. Am J Sports Med 37(5):909–916
5. Delzell PB, Schils JP, Recht MP (1996) Subtle fractures about the knee: innocuous-appearing yet indicative of significant internal derangement. AJR Am J Roentgenol 167(3):699–703
6. Dodds AL, Gupte CM, Neyret P et al (2011) Extra-articular techniques in anterior cruciate ligament reconstruction: a literature review. J Bone Joint Surg Br 93(11):1440–1448
7. Tashman S, Collon D, Anderson K (2004) Abnormal rotational knee motion during running after anterior cruciate ligament reconstruction. Am J Sports Med 32(4):975–983
8. Marcacci M, Zaffagnini S, Marcheggiani Muccioli GM et al (2011) Arthroscopic intra- and extra-articular anterior cruciate ligament reconstruction with gracilis and semitendinosus tendons: a review. Curr Rev Musculoskelet Med 4(2):73–77
9. Zaffagnini S, Signorelli C, Lopomo N et al (2012) Anatomic double-bundle and over-the-top single-bundle with additional extra-articular tenodesis: an in vivo quantitative assessment of knee laxity in two different ACL reconstructions. Knee Surg Sports Traumatol Arthrosc 20(1):153–159
10. Dejour D, Vasconcelos W, Bonin N (2013) Comparative study between mono-bundle bone-patellar tendon-bone, double-bundle hamstring and mono-bundle bone-patellar tendon-bone combined with a modified Lemaire extra-articular procedure in anterior cruciate ligament reconstruction. Int Orthop 37:193–199

11. Marcacci M, Zaffagnini S, Giordano G et al (2009) Anterior cruciate ligament reconstruction associated with extra-articular tenodesis: A prospective clinical and radiographic evaluation with 10- to 13-year follow-up. Am J Sports Med 37(4):707–714
12. Bignozzi S, Zaffagnini S, Lopomo N et al (2009) Does a lateral plasty control coupled translation during antero-posterior stress in single-bundle ACL reconstruction? An in vivo study. Knee Surg Sports Traumatol Arthrosc 17(1):65–70
13. Buda R, Ruffilli A, Di Caprio F (2013) Allograft salvage procedure in multiple-revision anterior cruciate ligament reconstruction. Am J Sports Med 41(2):402–410
14. Trojani C, Beaufils P, Burdin G (2012) Revision ACL reconstruction: influence of a lateral tenodesis. Knee Surg Sports Traumatol Arthrosc 20(8):1565–1570
15. Krackow KA, Brooks RL (1983) Optimization of knee ligament position for lateral extraarticular reconstruction. Am J Sports Med 11(5):293–302
16. Zaffagnini S, Klos TV, Bignozzi S (2010) Computer-assisted anterior cruciate ligament reconstruction: an evidence-based approach of the first 15 years. Arthroscopy 26(4):546–554
17. Colombet PD (2011) Navigated intra-articular ACL reconstruction with additional extra-articular tenodesis using the same hamstring graft. Knee Surg Sports Traumatol Arthrosc 19(3):384–389
18. Engebretsen L, Lew WD, Lewis JL et al (1990) The effect of an iliotibial tenodesis on intraarticular graft forces and knee joint motion. Am J Sports Med 18(2):169–176
19. Roth JH, Kennedy JC, Lockstadt H et al (1987) Intra-articular reconstruction of the anterior cruciate ligament with and without extra-articular supplementation by transfer of the biceps femoris tendon. J Bone Joint Surg Am 69(2):275–278
20. Strum GM, Fox JM, Ferkel RD et al (1989) Intraarticular versus intraarticular and extraarticular reconstruction for chronic anterior cruciate ligament instability. Clin Orthop Relat Res 245:188–198
21. Acquitter Y, Hulet C, Locker B et al (2003) Patellar tendon-bone autograft reconstruction of the anterior cruciate ligament for advanced-stage chronic anterior laxity: is an extra-articular plasty necessary? A prospective randomized study of 100 patients with five year follow-up. Rev Chir Orthop Reparatrice Appar Mot 89(5):413–422
22. Giraud B, Besse JL, Cladiere F et al (2006) Intra-articular reconstruction of the anterior cruciate ligament with and without extra-articular supplementation by quadricipital tendon plasty: seven-year follow-up. Rev Chir Orthop Reparatrice Appar Mot 92(8):788–797
23. Lerat JL, Chotel F, Besse JL et al (1998) The results after 10–16 years of the treatment of chronic anterior laxity of the knee using reconstruction of the anterior cruciate ligament with a patellar tendon graft combined with an external extra-articular reconstruction. Rev Chir Orthop Reparatrice Appar Mot 84(8):712–727
24. Zaffagnini S, Marcacci M, Lo Presti M et al (2006) Prospective and randomized evaluation of ACL reconstruction with three techniques: a clinical and radiographic evaluation at 5 years follow-up. Knee Surg Sports Traumatol Arthrosc 14(11):1060–1069
25. Monaco E, Labianca L, Conteduca F et al (2007) Double bundle or single bundle plus extraarticular tenodesis in ACL reconstruction? A CAOS study. Knee Surg Sports Traumatol Arthrosc 15(10):1168–1174

Combined PCL and Peripheral Instability

13

Rodrigo Maestu, Pablo Rainaudi, and Francisco Ciliberto

13.1 Introduction

The posterior cruciate ligament (PCL) is an intra-articular and extra-synovial ligament with a length that varies between 32 and 38 mm and with a surface in its transversal section that reaches 11 mm^2 [1, 2]. It has ample insertions in the medial femoral condyle and in the posterior tibial sector. PCL's footprint, both tibial and femoral, may triple its transversal section in surface [1].

Although it is a bundle of fibers which change their tension depending on the flexion degree of the knee, for better understanding of its function, it can be divided into an anterolateral band (AL), which has a larger size, and a posteromedial band (PM) [1–3].

Thereby, anatomic and biomechanical studies show that the AL band becomes tense in flexion with its maximum at 90° and that the PM band becomes tense in extension [1, 2]. Even though the latter is what bibliography accepts the most, there are in vivo biomechanical studies which show that both bands become tense as knee flexion increases [3].

There is also another synergic component with PCL which is the meniscofemoral ligaments. These are two unsteady ligaments [4] that are inserted into the posterior horn of the lateral meniscus and from there head toward the outer wall of the medial femoral condyle. One of them inserts in front of the PCL (Humphrey) and the other one behind it (Wrisberg). These have a secondary role in the posterior stabilization of the knee [1, 2].

PCL is the main stabilizer of the posterior tibial translation of the tibia. This function is more marked at 90° of knee flexion [1, 5]. Besides, it is also a safe stabilizer of external rotation [5].

R. Maestu, MD (✉) • P. Rainaudi, MD • F. Ciliberto, MD
CETEA (Center for the Study and Treatment of Joint Diseases),
Cervinio 4449, 9th floor, Caba, Buenos Aires 1625, Argentina
e-mail: rmaestu@intramed.net; pablorainaudi@yahoo.com.ar; franciliberto@hotmail.com

R. Rossi, F. Margheritini (eds.), *Knee Ligament Injuries*,
DOI 10.1007/978-88-470-5513-1_13, © Springer Verlag Italia 2014

PCL femoral insertion is elliptic and is 32 mm long, ending approximately at 3 mm proximal to the articular cartilage edge of the medial femoral condyle. The distal insertion is found in the posterior aspect of the tibia at 1–1.5 cm distal to the posterior edge of the tibia [2].

The main mechanism by which the PCL gets injured is due to an impact of anteroposterior direction at the proximal end of the tibia or due to a hyperextension mechanism.

PCL lesions are generally well tolerated. Patients rarely complain of instability episodes, but they complain more commonly about pain. This occurs predominantly in the internal or patellofemoral sector of the knee [6, 7]. In earlier times, this led to very controversial points of view concerning surgical treatment of PCL lesions.

Several biomechanical studies of the series of patients showed that the consequence of knee cinematic anomaly with PCL deficiency leads to articulation overload, mainly in the patellofemoral and medial tibiofemoral compartments together with arthritic degeneration [6, 7].

PCL reconstruction aims to restore the normal biomechanics of the knee to avoid these changes, although this aim is controversial [6].

13.2 Diagnosis of PCL and Combined Lesions

13.2.1 Physical Examination

Physical examination is very important, but in some acute cases, it may be difficult, even more with combined lesions.

You should rule out neurovascular lesions and, if you are not sure, order vascular studies (arteriography) and one consultation with a specialist. And you should also check soft tissue trauma.

On physical examination, knee posterior stability must be evaluated. The most representative semiologic maneuver is the posterior drawer.

The posterior tibial displacement allows us to classify PCL lesions in three grades: (1) displacement lower than 5 mm, (2) displacement between 6 and 10 mm, and (3) displacement higher than 10 mm [8].

Displacement can also be measured according to the relationship between the femur and tibia: (A) The anterior tibial edge displaces backward but remains anterior to the medial femoral condyle. (B) The anterior tibial edge displaces backward reaching the same level as the medial femoral condyle. (C) The anterior tibial edge displaces behind the medial femoral condyle.

Other semiologic maneuvers to assess posterior instability are Godfrey test and quad activation test.

It is important to take into account that PCL lesions almost always make part of a multiligament lesion. Therefore physical examination must be oriented toward detecting any other associated lesion [8].

If the knee has a posterior instability, it is routine to check the anterior cruciate ligament (ACL), medial collateral ligament (MCL), lateral collateral ligament (LCL), and both corners (posteromedial and posterolateral).

In general PCL grades 3 or C lesions are associated to a posterolateral corner lesion [8].

13.2.2 Complementary Studies

First of all we order X-rays. These are the routine views: anteroposterior weight bearing, lateral in 90°, and Merchant patella views. These should always be bilateral.

We rule out fractures or avulsions, and besides, in the lateral views, the posterior translation of the tibia from the femur can be seen. In chronic cases what can be seen is the condition of the medial and patellofemoral compartments; habitually in these cases, there is cartilage damage.

The other study we indicate is an MRI to assess ligaments and the whole knee: cartilage, meniscus, capsule, bone, etc.

13.3 Treatment

13.3.1 Posterior and Medial or Posteromedial Instability

The MCL has 2 separate structures: superficial MCL (sMCL) and deep MCL (dMCL) [9].

The posterior oblique ligament (POL) is a structure located posteriorly to the MCL. It runs from the semimembranosus tendon to the posterior medial aspect of the knee [10].

13.3.1.1 Acute Cases

A conservative treatment should always be indicated for PCL and MCL, except for fractures or avulsions. The PCL and MCL ligaments have healing power, and in many cases, the patient gains an adequate posterior and medial stabilization with a conservative treatment [11].

We indicate a brace in extension (with antepulsion of the calf) and crutches during 4–6 weeks, and then we evaluate the PCL and MCL with a physical examination and an MRI.

Following the above, we indicate surgical reconstruction either of PCL or of MCL or both. The surgical technique is the same as in chronic cases.

First we prefer to perform PCL and then MCL reconstruction all at once.

13.3.1.2 Chronic Cases

When patients come to the clinic 4–6 weeks after the lesion occurred.

Grafts

They depend on each individual patient. In people below 35 years of age, we prefer to use hamstring tendon autografts for PCL and allografts (anterior tibial tendon) for MCL. In patients over 35 years, we use allografts for everything (two anterior tibial tendons).

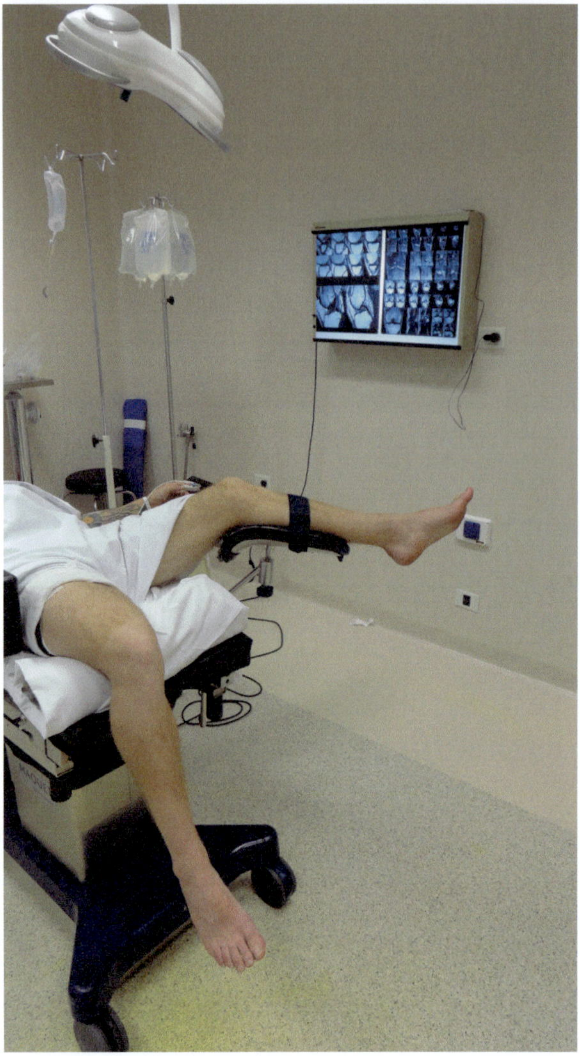

Fig. 13.1 Position of the patient for a PCL surgery. Left leg holder giving room to work through the posteromedial portal

Surgical Technique

The position of the patient on the OR table is fundamental. Firstly, the knee should be in 90° with the possibility to bend it in full flexion. Next, is to have a lateral support to be able to perform a knee valgus to explore the medial compartment. Lastly, the other hip must be in flexion and in abduction and the other leg away from the OR table so as to work easily through the posteromedial portal (Fig. 13.1).

In these cases we use pneumatic tourniquet. If the surgery takes over 100 min, it is necessary to discontinue the pneumatic tourniquet for 20 min and then use it again. Concerning the portals, we usually use 3: anterolateral, anteromedial, and posteromedial.

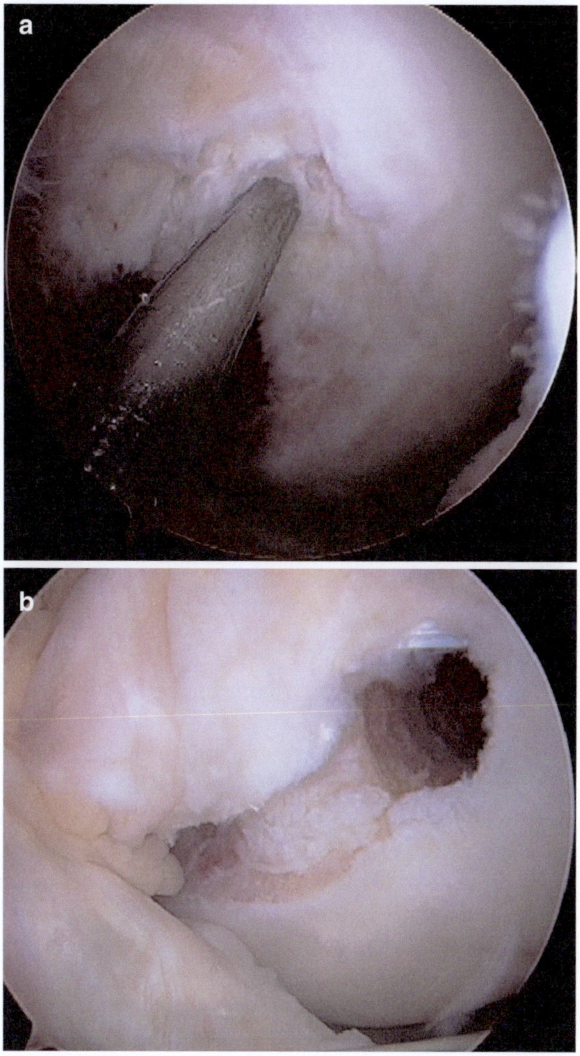

Fig. 13.2 (**a**) Guide pin in PM femoral bundle location for an augmentation procedure. (**b**) Bleeding bone bed in the outer wall of the medial femoral condyle for the PCL graft. Right knee

The first step is to perform the PCL arthroscopic reconstruction and afterward the medial reconstruction in the same surgical time.

After examining and treating meniscal and cartilage lesions of the medial, lateral, and patellofemoral compartments, we perform the PCL femoral anatomic tunnel inside out.

If patient has an intact band or a remnant of PCL, we always preserve it and perform an augmentation.

We use a femoral aimer (through the anterolateral portal) to place the exact anatomic tunnel position of the ligament, and we check the pin position through the same portal to be sure of the correct position. We try to reconstruct the AL band (Fig. 13.2a).

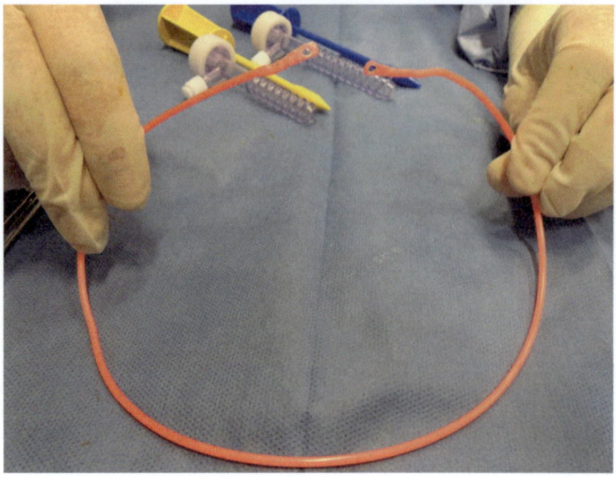

Fig. 13.3 Homemade plastic device to raise the PCL graft

Regarding femoral tunnel size, for PCL we use a length of 25 mm and the width is the same as the graft, usually 8–9 mm.

Then with a shaver or rasp, we make a bleeding bone bed in the medial notch where the PCL graft will be placed (Fig. 13.2b).

When we have the PCL femoral tunnel ready, we perform the posteromedial portal and insert an 8 mm cannula in. And then we begin to clean the posterior tibia with a shaver or radiofrequency. We try to expose 20 mm of the posterior tibia to be able to locate the PCL guide easily. It is very useful to have a reliable and accurate PCL guide and curved curettes to protect the pin exit not to damage the knee posterior structures. It is a very good maneuver to use a curved rasp to make a bleeding bone bed in the posterior tibia where the PCL graft will lay. We use a guide that marks how deep we are in the posterior tibia, and as the tip guide is wide, it stops the pin from going farther and damaging the posterior neurovascular structures. For greater safety we can also use a special device with the guide so as to keep the pin from going further than the guide tip.

We raise the PCL graft through the tibial tunnel to the femur. It is very useful to have some malleable material as a plastic with a hole in both ends to do it (Fig. 13.3). To help the advancement of the graft, we use the trocar of the scope through the posteromedial portal as a pulley. In the proximal PCL graft, we make a suture with 2 cm baseball stitches for better screw fixation. We fix the proximal end of the graft with a 7 and 25 mm interferential BioScrew with the knee in 90°. Lastly we fix the distal PCL graft with a BioScrew which is one or two numbers higher than the graft and 30 mm long; the knee must be in 90° flexion with an antepulsion of the calf (because we are reconstructing the AL band).

Concerning medial or posteromedial instability, we prefer to reconstruct the sMCL and the POL. In cases when the patient has no posteromedial instability, we only perform the sMCL.

As regards posteromedial instability, we perform only one tunnel in the femur, 0.5 mm posterior and 0.5 mm proximal to the medial epicondyle [12], for proximal

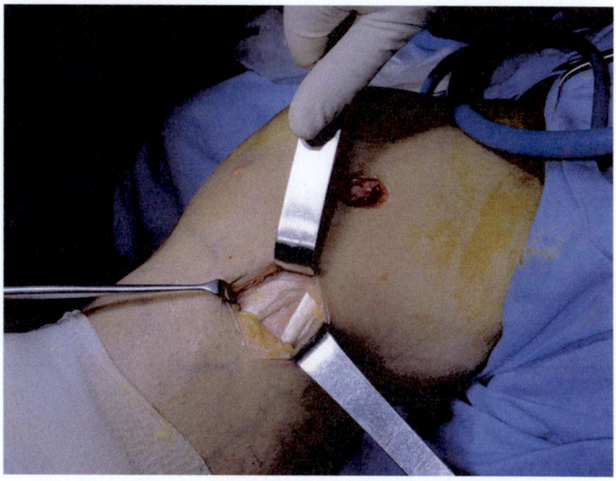

Fig. 13.4 Final reconstruction of the sMCL and POL. Right knee

insertion of the sMCL and POL. The tunnel diameter size depends on the graft (usually 8 or 9 mm for a double anterior tibial allograft), but its length is always 30 mm. The proximal skin incision is approximately 20 mm long.

In tibia, for the sMCL we perform a tunnel in the anterior face of the tibia 60 mm distal to the knee joint line whose size depends on the graft (single anterior tibial allograft) and which runs through the whole tibia. For the POL we insert a 5 mm bioabsorbable anchor, with 2 sutures, 15 mm distal to the knee joint line and as far back as possible from the tibial anterior face. The distal skin incision depends on the patient, but if we have harvested hamstring tendons for the PCL, we use an oblique incision of 30–50 mm for the entire procedure.

We pass the graft underneath the semimembranosus attached to the periosteum.

In the femur, we fix the graft with an interferential BioScrew, which has the same diameter as the tunnel and is 30 mm long. We fix the sMCL with a 25 mm long BioScrew in 30° of knee flexion, respecting the same diameter as the tunnel, and if necessary, we add a staple. The last fixation is the distal POL, in full extension with the two reinforced sutures of the anchor (Fig. 13.4).

Post-op

Immobilization should be in full extension, with a brace and partial weight bearing using crutches 6–8 weeks.

13.3.2 Posterior and Lateral or Posterolateral Instability

The posterolateral corner is a complex structure which contributes to knee stability.

The most important structures are the lateral collateral ligament (LCL) or fibular collateral ligament, the popliteus tendon, the popliteus fibular ligament (PFL), and the posterolateral capsule [13, 14].

A specific maneuver to assess posterolateral instability is varus stress in full extension and in 30° of knee flexion.

Others are dial test, posterolateral drawer test, recurvatum test, and inverse pivot shift test. It is always advisable to perform them bilaterally. If in the dial test the comparative external rotation is higher than 10°, in 30° and 90°, it shows that PCL and posterolateral structures are torn. But if in 90° the difference is lower than 10°, it shows that the PCL is intact.

13.3.2.1 Acute Cases

In these cases we indicate surgical treatment at the moment of diagnosis. We perform open surgery in the posterolateral corner. We repair everything as much as we can: LCL, popliteus tendon, FPL, and capsule. And we always add an LCL and PFL reconstruction with an allograft (anterior tibial tendon). We reconstruct it with a tunnel in the fibula's head from anterior to posterior and from inferior to superior, the same size as the graft. Be aware of the peroneal nerve that passes 20 mm distal to the proximal tip of the fibula; we always look for it to know where it is and to protect it, but we try not to touch it (Fig. 13.5a). We pass the graft through the fibula and insert the reconstruction in the femur between insertions of the proximal LCL and the popliteus tendon. We fix it with 2 BioScrews: in the femur, they are of the same diameter as the graft and 30 mm long, and, in the fibula with a small screw, generally 7×20 mm. When we fix the reconstruction, the knee has to be in 30° of flexion with a slight valgus.

Following the above, we perform surgical reconstruction of PCL at the same time. We prefer autograft hamstring tendons for young patients (under 35–40 years) and anterior tibial allograft for older patients (over 35–40 years).

13.3.2.2 Chronic Cases

We prefer to reconstruct the PCL and the LCL or LCL plus posterolateral corner in only one surgery.

Grafts

Formerly we described what we prefer for PCL. Concerning LCL and posterolateral corner, we like allografts for both (anterior tibial tendons).

Surgical Technique

We have already explained PCL technique above.

We perform the PCL reconstruction and, afterward in the same surgical time, the LCL and, when necessary, the posterolateral corner reconstruction.

To reconstruct just the LCL, we perform two small incisions: one across the fibula head (50 mm long) and the other one in the femur (15 mm long). Formerly we described the technique.

If the patient has a posterolateral and rotational instability, we reconstruct the popliteus tendon, the LCL, and the popliteus fibular tendon (the last two have been described before), and we perform a curved incision and look for the peroneal nerve, but we try not to touch it (Fig. 13.5b).

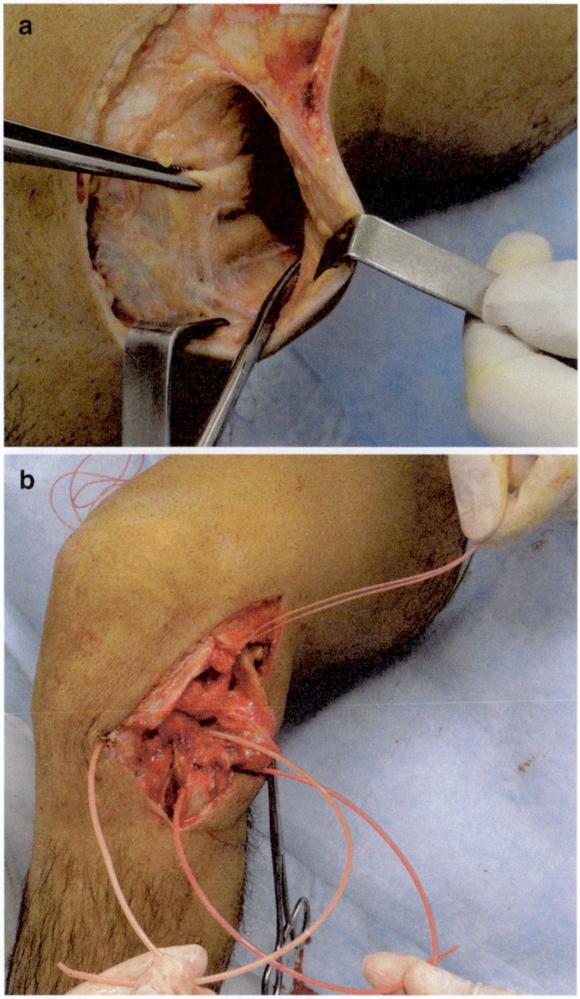

Fig. 13.5 (**a**) Biceps tendon and the peroneal nerve behind it. (**b**) Posterolateral reconstruction showing femoral tunnels, the popliteus tendon tunnel, and the fibular tunnel all ready to start graft pass

The popliteus reconstruction is through a tibial tunnel, beginning 20–30 mm distal to the knee joint from the medial tibia if we have harvested the hamstring tendons or from the lateral tibia if we use an allograft. The tunnel finishes in the posterolateral corner of the tibia; it is important to protect the pin exit with a curette prior to making the tunnel. The femoral tunnel comes before the LCL insertion (10 mm anterior), both in an anatomic position. Remember to pass the popliteus reconstruction below the LCL.

We fix the reconstruction with two BioScrews: in the femur their diameter size is the same as the graft and 30 mm long; and in the tibia, their diameter size is one or two more mm than the graft and 30 mm long; if necessary we add a staple. We fix the reconstruction in 30° of knee flexion.

If the patient has a varus deformity, it is important to evaluate, in chronic cases, the indication of a possible valgus osteotomy.

Post-op
Immobilization has to be in full extension with a brace and partial weight bearing with the use of crutches 6–8 weeks.

13.3.3 Posterior, Medial or Posteromedial, and Lateral or Posterolateral Instability

The last combination would be lesions of PCL, MCL (with or without posteromedial corner), and LCL (with or without posterolateral corner).

We have already described all the techniques above.

First of all we check and treat neurovascular and soft lesions. We indicate crutches and immobilization for at least 2 weeks, and then we assess all the structures.

13.3.3.1 Surgery

We make a medial and lateral corner repair plus reconstruction with allografts (we prefer anterior tibial tendons), and later, at the same time, if the patient has posterior instability, we perform a PCL arthroscopy reconstruction with an allograft (anterior tibial). We prefer to begin with the lateral side.

Conclusion

We think PCL and MCL have healing power; for that reason, our first option, of course ruling out neurovascular and soft tissue lesions, in acute cases is to try a conservative treatment for at least 4 weeks, and then we evaluate the patient again. Indications for early repair and reconstruction are irreducible dislocations, dysvascular limbs, open injuries, and fractures or avulsions.

In chronic cases or when the capsule is healthy, first we prefer to perform the arthroscopy time, to avoid extravasation of fluid into the compartments which runs the risk of compartment syndromes.

Regarding tips and tricks, with PCL, our advice is as follows: use soft tissue grafts, femur tunnel inside out before tibial tunnel; keep the remnant as intact as possible; have a good vision through the posteromedial portal; help biology performing blood bone bed where the graft will be placed; use the right PCL guide; have a correct device to raise the graft through the tibial tunnel; and indicate a very conservative rehab.

Concerning multiligamentous injuries always perform reconstructions besides repairs: in posterolateral corners with LCL and the FPL reconstructions (with a tibial anterior tendon allograft), and in the posteromedial corner with sMCL reconstruction (with a tibial anterior tendon allograft).

And lastly, the most important thing is to know the knee anatomy.

References

1. Voos JE, Mauro CS, Wente T, Warren RF, Wickiewicz TL (2012) Posterior cruciate ligament anatomy, biomechanics, and outcomes. Am J Sports Med 40(1):222–231
2. Insall JN, Scott NW (2007) Anatomía. In: Rodilla, 3rd edn. Marbán, Madrid, pp 13–74
3. Papannagari R, DeFrate LE, Nha KW, Moses JM, Moussa M, Gill TJ, Li G (2007) Function of posterior cruciate ligament bundles during in vivo knee flexion. Am J Sports Med 35(9):1507–1512
4. Amis AA, Gupte CM, Bull AMJ, Edwards A (2006) Anatomy of the posterior cruciate ligament and the meniscofemoral ligaments. Knee Surg Sports Traumatol Arthrosc 14(3):257–263
5. Insall JN, Scott NW (2007) Lesiones del ligamento cruzado posterior. In: Rodilla, 3rd edn. Marbán, Madrid, pp 879–891
6. Gill TJ, DeFrate LE, Wang C, Carey CT, Zayontz S, Zarins B, Li G (2004) The effect of posterior cruciate ligament reconstruction on patellofemoral contact pressures in the knee joint under simulated muscle loads. Am J Sports Med 32(1):109–115
7. Li G, Papannagari R, Li M, Bingham J, Nha KW, Allred D, Gill T (2008) Effect of posterior cruciate ligament deficiency on in vivo translation and rotation of the knee during weightbearing flexion. Am J Sports Med 36(3):474–479
8. Wind WM, Bergfeld JA, Parker RD (2004) Evaluation and treatment of posterior cruciate ligament injuries revisited. Am J Sports Med 32(7):1765–1775
9. LaPrade RF, Engebretsen AH, Ly TV, Johansen S, Wentorf FA, Engebretsen L (2007) The anatomy of the medial part of the knee. J Bone Joint Surg 89(9):2000–2010
10. Sims WF, Jacobson KE (2004) The posteromedial corner of the knee medial-sided injury patterns revisited. Am J Sports Med 32(2):337–345
11. Shelbourne KD, Carr DR (2003) Combined anterior and posterior cruciate and medial collateral ligament injury: nonsurgical and delayed surgical treatment. Instr Course Lect 52:413
12. Wijdicks CA, Griffith CJ, Johansen S, Engebretsen L, LaPrade RF (2010) Injuries to the medial collateral ligament and associated medial structures of the knee. J Bone Joint Surg 92(5):1266–1280
13. LaPrade RF, Ly TV, Wentorf FA, Engebretsen L (2003) The posterolateral attachments of the knee a qualitative and quantitative morphologic analysis of the fibular collateral ligament, popliteus tendon, popliteofibular ligament, and lateral gastrocnemius tendon. Am J Sports Med 31(6):854–860
14. Ranalletta A, Ranalletta M, Rossi W, Vieta R, Paoletta R, Garcia Hamilton P (2011) Angulo posteroexterno de la rodilla: anatomía aplicada a la técnica quirurgica; Posterolateral corner of the knee: surgical anatomy. Arthrosc (B Aires) 18(3):104–107

Treatment for Acute Knee Dislocations 14

Alexander E. Weber and Jon K. Sekiya

14.1 Introduction

Acute knee dislocations are infrequent injuries; however, the sequelae may be quite severe and potentially limb threatening. Furthermore, the incidence of acute knee dislocations has been rising. The increased incidence may be a by-product of escalated involvement in contact athletics coupled with an increased participation in nontraditional sporting and recreational activities such as the riding of motorbikes, snowmobiles, and all-terrain vehicles. Although there is a rise in the incidence of knee dislocations, there is a lag in high-level-of-evidence studies from which a consensus statement on the treatment of these injuries may be derived. However, from the available prospective studies and systematic reviews in conjunction with our senior author's expert opinion, we have compiled this guide to the treatment of the acutely dislocated knee.

14.2 Definition

The definition of a knee dislocation is most simply the complete disruption of the tibiofemoral articulation. Following the acute event, the knee may spontaneously reduce or it may remain dislocated. The dislocation event is always coupled with a multiligamentous knee injury of variable degree. The definition of a multiligamentous knee injury is the rupture of two or more of the major ligaments/ligamentous complexes of the knee: anterior cruciate ligament (ACL), posterior cruciate ligament (PCL), medial collateral ligament (MCL), posteromedial corner (posterior oblique

A.E. Weber, MD • J.K. Sekiya, MD (✉)
Orthopaedic Surgery, University of Michigan,
MedSport, Lobby A, 24 Frank Lloyd Wright Dr., Ann Arbor, MI 48106, USA
e-mail: alexweb@med.umich.edu; sekiya@hotmail.com;
schauer@umich.edu; schauer@med.umich.edu

R. Rossi, F. Margheritini (eds.), *Knee Ligament Injuries*,
DOI 10.1007/978-88-470-5513-1_14, © Springer Verlag Italia 2014

ligament, semimembranosus expansions, oblique popliteal ligament; PMC), lateral collateral ligament (LCL), or posterolateral corner (LCL, popliteus, and popliteofibular ligament; PLC). Most commonly, an acute dislocation results in rupture of both cruciates (ACL and PCL) and one additional ligamentous structure [1–5]. Less frequently, but described in the literature, is the occurrence of an acute knee dislocation with a resultant ligamentous injury that spares the PCL, the so-called PCL-intact knee dislocation [4, 6, 7].

14.3 Epidemiology and Mechanism

Knee dislocation is a relatively rare injury, constituting 0.02–0.2 % of all orthopedic injuries [8–11]. However, some authors suggest the incidence of knee dislocation may be significantly higher because the vast majority of dislocations spontaneously reduce prior to hospital presentation. The patient demographic tends to be young males, with a male-to-female ratio of 4 to 1. These injuries are most frequently (50 %) caused by a high-velocity mechanism such as a motor vehicle accident, motorcycle collision, or all-terrain vehicle. One of the most typical mechanisms of dislocation in the high-energy cohort is a posteriorly directed force on the tibia as it strikes the dashboard or steering wheel during a crash [1, 12]. High-energy knee dislocations are present as a component of the polytraumatized patient in 14–44 % of cases. Although the likelihood of bilateral knee dislocations is quite low at 5 %, the rate of open injury associated with a knee dislocation ranges from 5 to 17 % in the literature [13].

An additional one-third of knee dislocations are secondary to low-velocity sports injuries, while one-tenth of all dislocations are due to a fall [14]. Shelbourne presented a case series of low-velocity knee dislocations secondary to football, wrestling, and running injuries [14]. The characteristic mechanism of injury in the athletic knee dislocation is a contact or collision that forces the knee into hyperextension combined with excessive varus or valgus force. It is important for the team physician to distinguish this mechanism from that of an isolated ACL rupture, which is typically sustained via a noncontact injury mechanism. An additional mechanism of injury, as described in the literature, is the "spontaneous" dislocation in the morbidly obese patient [15, 16].

14.4 Classification

The original knee dislocation classification system was proposed by Kennedy in 1963 and was purely descriptive in nature based upon the direction of the dislocation [12]. The five categories based on direction were anterior, posterior, medial, lateral, and rotatory. Based on direction, anterior dislocation is the most common followed by posterior dislocation. Rotatory dislocation is the least common [12, 17].

Table 14.1 Knee dislocation anatomic classification system

	Anatomic classification of knee dislocation
KD-I	Single cruciate torn (ACL or PCL)
KD-II	Bicruciate tears (ACL and PCL)
KD-III	Bicruciate tears plus MCL or LCL/PLC
KD-IV	ACL, PCL, MCL, LCL/PLC tears
KD-V	All ligaments with an associated fracture

Adapted from Schenck [18]
ACL anterior cruciate ligament, *PCL* posterior cruciate ligament, *MCL* medial collateral ligament, *LCL* lateral collateral ligament, *PLC* posterolateral corner

A limitation of this system was that it could not be used in cases of dislocation followed by spontaneous reduction. Schenck proposed a modified classification system that accounts for the pattern of injury and is thus anatomically based (Table 14.1) [18]. The anatomic classification of knee dislocations helps to guide treatment and provides a "common language" to compare outcomes for different injury patterns and across different studies in the literature.

14.5 Initial Evaluation and Management

Identification of a knee dislocation is relatively easy if the knee remains dislocated at the time of presentation; however, a high index of suspicion is necessary in cases of dislocation followed by spontaneous reduction in the field. The clinician should be highly suspicious for knee dislocation if there is misalignment of the affected lower extremity, deformity of the knee, massive soft tissue swelling, or disproportionate pain (Fig. 14.1a). The absence of a joint effusion may be a misleading and false sense of comfort as high-energy dislocations can result in capsular damage, which will allow the knee effusion to diffuse into the surrounding soft tissue.

Patients presenting with knee trauma should be treated like any other traumatized patient, and the first step should always be implementation of the Advanced Trauma Life Support (ATLS) protocol [19]. Following ATLS protocol, and assuming the patient is without more pressing injuries, a dislocated knee should be reduced. In cases of high-energy knee dislocations, a portable "spot shot" radiograph of the knee should be taken prior to reduction to confirm the absence of major fractures. If fractures of the distal femur or proximal tibia are present, the clinician may opt to reduce the knee if the fractures appear relatively stable. In cases of low-energy trauma, such as knee dislocations sustained on the playing field, immediate reduction should be attempted prior to imaging studies. Post-reduction radiographs should always be obtained to confirm a concentric reduction of the tibiofemoral articulation (Fig. 14.1b). The knee should be initially inspected for any evidence of an open injury that would necessitate a formal irrigation and debridement in the operating room.

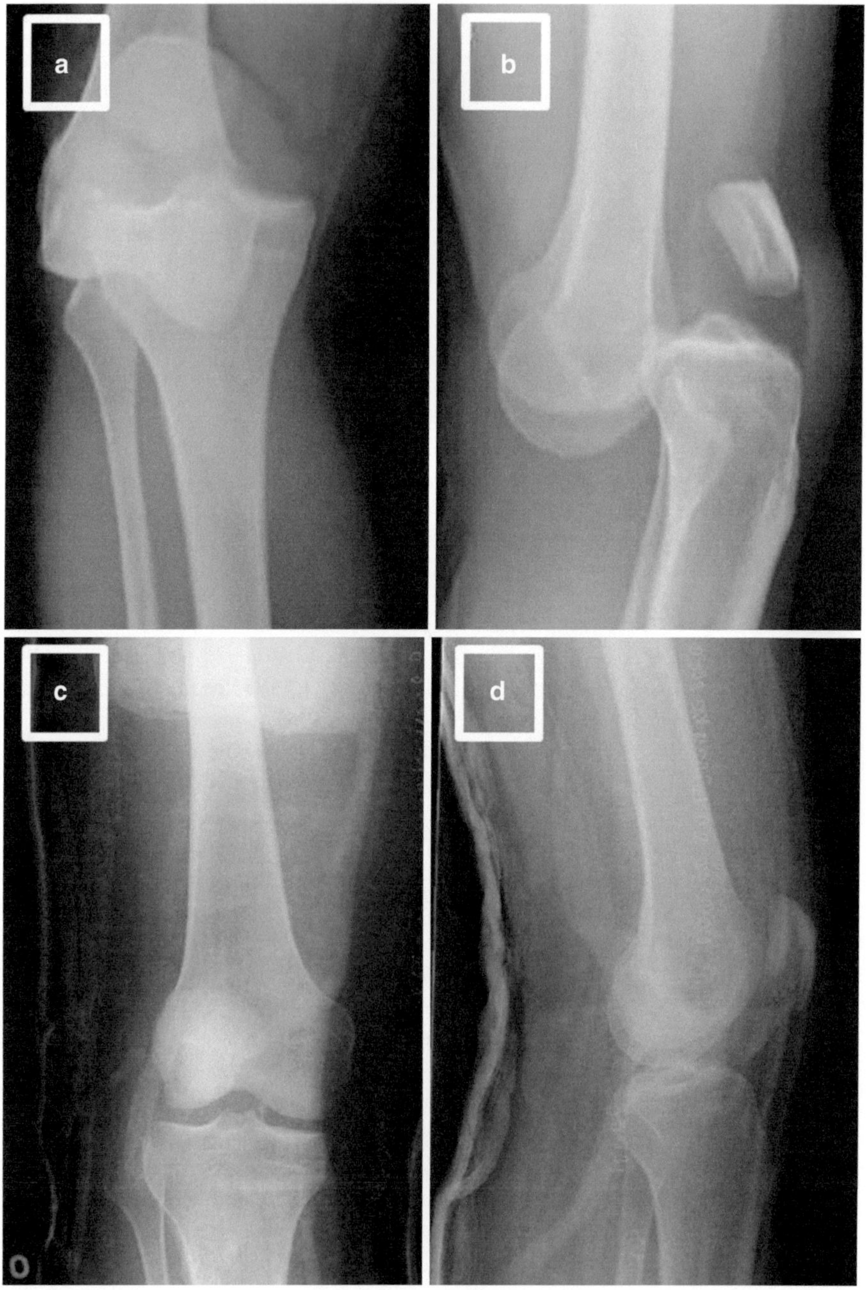

Fig. 14.1 (**a**) Anteroposterior and (**b**) lateral radiographs demonstrating an anterior knee dislocation. (**c**) Anteroposterior and (**d**) lateral radiographs demonstrating an adequate reduction of previous anterior knee dislocation

14.6 Vascular Evaluation and Management

Following confirmed reduction of the knee, a thorough vascular examination should be completed. The incidence of popliteal artery injury associated with knee dislocation has been reported to range from 4.8 to 65 %, with posterior knee dislocations having the highest rate of injury [8, 20, 21]. Vascular injuries are not solely associated with high-energy knee dislocations. Low-energy and spontaneous knee dislocations can cause vascular occlusion or intimal tearing [17, 22]. This examination should begin with inspection of the color, temperature, and capillary refill of the affected leg. Distal arterial flow in the dorsalis pedis, posterior tibial, and peroneal arteries should be interrogated first manually and secondarily with Doppler ultrasound if necessary. The clinician should be cognizant that a normal physical examination and palpable distal pulses do not exclude serious vascular injury, such as an intimal tear to the popliteal artery [23]. The ankle-brachial index (ABI) should be calculated using Doppler ultrasound and a blood pressure cuff if there is any concern for the vascular status. The ratio of systolic blood pressure in the affected ankle is compared to the unaffected upper arm. In a knee dislocation cohort, Mills reported 100 % sensitivity, specificity, and positive predictive value of a significant arterial injury requiring surgical attention if the ABI is below 0.90 [23]. Absent pulses or diminished ABIs are indications for involvement of a vascular surgeon. It is important to involve vascular surgery colleagues in an expeditious fashion, as warm ischemia time of greater than 6–8 h is associated with a higher rate of amputation [17, 24]. Additional studies or interventions that are frequently requested by a vascular surgeon include computed tomography angiogram (CTA) and formal angiography (Fig. 14.2). An abnormal CTA will necessitate a formal angiogram with either endovascular or open vascular intervention. At our institution a formal angiogram with or without intervention is accompanied by external fixation performed by an orthopedic surgeon to stabilize the knee, provide access for additional vascular procedures (the external fixation eliminates the need for a splint), and permit serial examinations of the affected limb postoperatively.

14.7 Neurologic Evaluation and Management

The incidence of nerve injury with acute knee dislocation is approximately 20 % [12, 25]. The most commonly injured nerve is the common peroneal nerve rather than the tibial nerve. The explanation for the higher incidence of peroneal nerve injury is its anatomic course adjacent to the proximal fibula, the decreased compliance compared to the tibial nerve, and the mechanism of knee dislocation. Lateral and posterolateral dislocations can significantly stretch the peroneal nerve. To identify these injuries, the clinician should perform an initial tactile exam of the patient's sensation in all nerve distributions of the lower extremity. Graded motor strength with ankle dorsiflexion, ankle plantar flexion, ankle inversion, ankle eversion, and

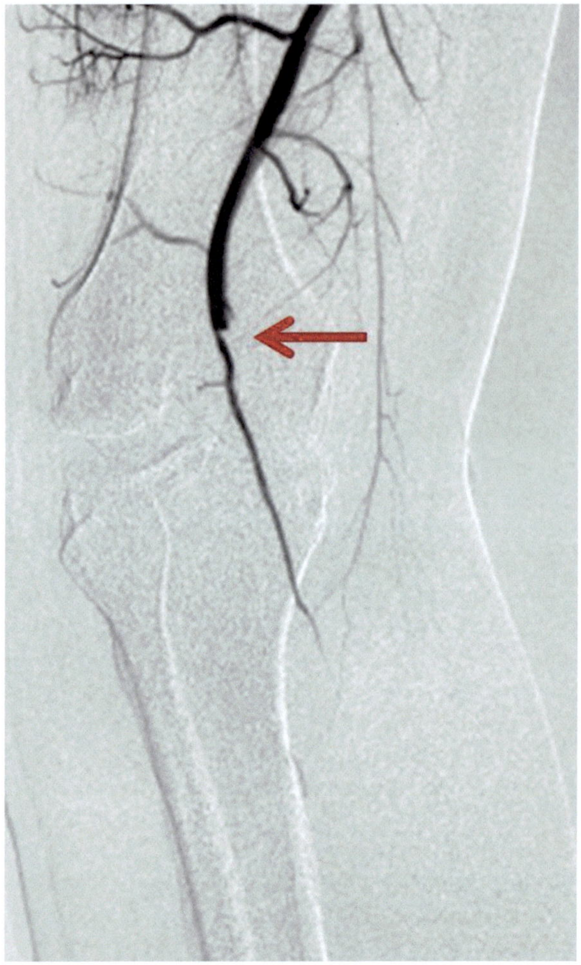

Fig. 14.2 Representative angiogram demonstrating lack of significant distal flow beyond the popliteal hiatus (popliteal artery) secondary to a knee dislocation. *Arrow* indicates significant obstruction

great toe dorsiflexion should be documented. There is no acute treatment for neurologic deficits following knee dislocation, and the overall prognosis for neurologic recovery remains low [26]. Chronic neurologic injuries such as foot drop may be treated with an ankle foot orthosis or a posterior tibial tendon transfer.

14.8 Ligamentous Evaluation

A thorough ligamentous examination should be performed on all patients with a suspected knee dislocation. The initial examination may be limited due to pain, hematoma, or associated injuries; however, gross laxity or instability should be documented to the best of the examiner's abilities. It is important for the examiner to comment on the integrity of the main ligamentous stabilizers, including the ACL, PCL, MCL, LCL, and PLC. A brief review of the basic ligamentous examination is presented here.

The anterior drawer and Lachman examinations are performed to evaluate for laxity in the ACL, the latter of which is considered the more accurate maneuver [27]. Both examinations grade the magnitude of anterior-posterior (A-P) translation of the tibia in relation to the femur and the presence or absence of a firm endpoint of that motion. The presence of an ACL tear is typically apparent due to increased translation and a lack of a firm endpoint compared to the contralateral knee. A caveat for these maneuvers in the setting of an acute knee dislocation is that it may be difficult or impossible to flex the affected knee to 90° to perform the anterior drawer test secondary to pain, swelling, or fracture. In addition, both examination maneuvers take advantage of the normal anatomic resting position of the tibia in relation to the femur as the "starting point" for the examination of the magnitude of A-P translation. Typically the tibia lies anterior to the femur; however, if the PCL is disrupted, the tibial "starting point" may be translated posteriorly rendering the motion appreciated difficult to associate with ACL laxity rather than PCL laxity.

The third ACL examination maneuver is the pivot-shift test. This is the senior author's preferred test for grading ACL laxity during an examination under anesthesia; however, it is difficult to perform on the awake patient due to the inability to control hip and leg position. In addition, the pivot-shift test requires an intact iliotibial band (ITB) for accurate results. In the acute knee dislocation, there may be tearing or disruption of the ITB. Lastly, pain, swelling, and fracture are additional reasons this examination maneuver may be difficult to perform in the setting of an acute knee dislocation.

The PCL may be evaluated by assessing the posterior sag and the posterior drawer. The posterior sag test, performed with the knee and hip flexed to 90°, evaluates the position of the proximal tibia in relation to the distal femoral condyles. In the presence of a PCL tear, the proximal tibia will sag (posterior translation) relative to the distal femoral condyles as compared to the contralateral side. The posterior drawer test is performed in 90° of flexion by applying a posteriorly directed force on the proximal tibia with the thumbs on the joint line to quantify the distance of posterior translation. A grade III injury (greater than 10 mm of posterior translation) indicates a combined PCL and PLC injury [28].

Collateral ligament testing is performed with valgus (MCL) and varus (LCL) force on the knee. The testing is performed with the knee in 30° of flexion to isolate the collateral ligaments. The test is then repeated in full knee extension. Laxity at both 30° of flexion and full extension suggests disruption of additional structures. On the lateral side, laxity with varus stress in full extension suggests injury to the cruciate ligaments and the PLC in addition to the LCL [29]. On the medial side, laxity with valgus stress in full extension suggests injury to the cruciate ligaments and medial capsule in addition to the MCL.

The PMC is examined with maneuvers that place external rotation stress with the knee in various degrees of flexion. These tests help define the degree of anteromedial rotatory instability. The most common test is performed with the knee in 30° of flexion. A valgus stress is imposed while the foot is externally rotated [30, 31]. If this test elicits an increase in anteromedial external rotation as compared to the contralateral side, then a PMC injury has been sustained. In addition, if a combined PMC-PCL injury has been sustained, the magnitude of posterior translation of the tibia in the posterior drawer test will be exaggerated or unchanged with internal rotation of the tibia. In a PCL-deficient knee with an intact PMC, the magnitude of posterior tibial translation with the tibia internally rotated during the posterior drawer will be diminished [32, 33].

The PLC can be directly assessed with the dial test. The structures interrogated with this test include the LCL, popliteus tendon, and popliteofibular ligament [34]. With the patient prone, the knees are flexed to 30° and a symmetric, external rotation force is placed on both feet. The thigh-foot angle is measured and the test is again repeated at 90° of knee flexion. A difference in thigh-foot angle of greater than 10° side to side is considered a positive test. An increased thigh-foot angle at 30° of knee flexion but not at 90° is consistent with an isolated PLC injury, while increased thigh-foot angle at both 30 and 90° of knee flexion is consistent with a combined PCL and PLC injury. An isolated increase in thigh-foot angle at 90° of knee flexion suggests an injury to the PCL. The examiner should also be aware that increased thigh-foot angle rotation at 30 and 90° of knee flexion may signify an injury to the anteromedial aspect of the knee rather than the PLC [35].

14.9 Diagnostic Imaging

Radiographs of the knee in two planes (anteroposterior and lateral) should be performed to characterize the direction of dislocation (Fig. 14.1a, b). Initial radiographs are also important to assess for associated fractures, either large osseous injuries to the tibial plateau and distal femur or subtle fractures such as a Segond fracture or PCL avulsion. As mentioned previously, in low-velocity knee dislocations (sports injuries), a reduction should be attempted prior to the initial radiographs and ideally on the field if trained medical personnel are present. This is due to the low likelihood of significant fractures. However, in high-velocity knee dislocations (e.g., automobile accidents), the likelihood of significant fractures is much greater and thus plain radiographs should be performed prior to a reduction attempt. In either scenario, post-reduction radiographs should be obtained to confirm a concentric reduction (Fig. 14.1c, d). If there is concern for a PCL injury, stress radiographs of the bilateral knees may be performed with the knees flexed 80° and weight applied to the anterior tibia [36]. Stress radiographs may be more appropriate in the preoperative planning phase rather than acutely following a knee dislocation.

Once the knee is stabilized and vascular injuries have been ruled out, a computed tomography (CT) scan may be appropriate if fractures are present, and a magnetic resonance image (MRI) should be obtained to assess the extent of the ligamentous injury (Fig. 14.3). The MRI will also assist with preoperative planning in the case of damage to the chondral surfaces, menisci, and capsule. Bone bruising is common following acute knee dislocation and present 75 % of the time [37], while 25 % of

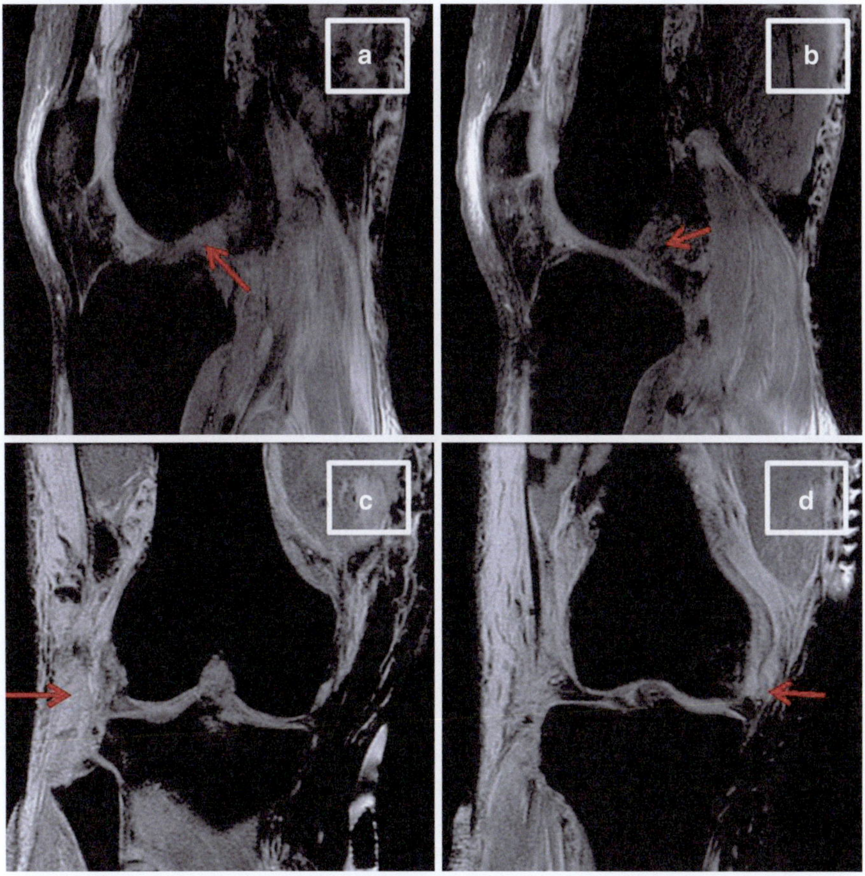

Fig. 14.3 (**a**) Sagittal magnetic resonance image (MRI) with *arrow* demonstrating complete disruption of the anterior cruciate ligament. (**b**) Sagittal MRI with *arrow* demonstrating complete disruption of the posterior cruciate ligament. (**c**) Coronal MRI with *arrow* demonstrating disruption of the lateral collateral ligament and posterolateral corner. (**d**) Coronal MRI with *arrow* demonstrating disruption of the medial collateral ligament

knee dislocations have concomitant meniscal injuries [37]. Furthermore, if fractures accompany the knee dislocation, the timing of MRI is crucial. Obtaining an MRI in the early phase of treatment, prior to open reduction and internal fixation of fractures, facilitates evaluation of ligamentous integrity without being obscured by the signal artifact of implanted hardware.

14.10 Initial Treatment

The initial care for a knee dislocation is dictated by a number of factors, including the open injury status, neurovascular status, fracture status, and ability to reduce the knee. If the dislocation is reduced, there is no fracture or open injury, and there is no concern for neurovascular compromise, then initial treatment may consist of a long-leg splint in 20° of knee flexion, lower extremity elevation, and serial neurovascular examinations. Twenty degrees of knee flexion is classically taught as the position for long-leg splinting; however, it is our experience that maintaining the knee in flexion for more than 3–5 days may compromise the ability to restore full extension long term. The treating surgeon should be cognizant of this during the initial management. If the knee dislocation is complicated by significant femoral condyle or tibial plateau fractures, an open injury, or a vascular injury or the knee is irreducible, then the complicating factor should be addressed in the operating room. Each of these complicating factors should also prompt the treating surgeon to consider concomitant application of external fixation rather than a splint at the conclusion of the operating room session. Stabilization of the dislocated knee with external fixation should also be considered in cases initially treated in a splint but with post-splinting films that demonstrate persistent tibiofemoral subluxation. Two important considerations when placing an external fixator following knee dislocation are that the hardware should be MRI compatible and the knee-spanning pins should be safely outside the knee joint and sufficiently away from future graft tunnel or fixation hardware sites. This "safe zone" for pin placement is roughly 10 cm proximal and distal to the knee joint line [38]. Lastly, if there is any clinical concern for compartment syndrome preoperatively or intraoperatively, the treating surgeon should have a low threshold for performing fasciotomies.

14.11 Definitive Treatment Considerations

Historically, the mainstay of knee dislocation definitive treatment was immobilization in plaster casts. However, as longitudinal clinical studies emerged, it became clear that patients sustaining knee dislocations and undergoing nonoperative treatment went on to develop persistent knee instability and had poor long-term functionality [39–42]. Recent studies suggest considerable benefit from surgical treatment [12, 21, 39, 41–45]. A recent systematic review comparing operative versus nonoperative treatments for multiligament knee injuries found significantly higher International Knee Documentation Committee (IKDC) scores, improved return-to-work rate, and higher rates of return to sport for patients in the cohort that underwent surgical treatment [44]. Dedmond and Almekinders [39] performed a meta-analysis of differences between operative and nonoperative treatment of acute knee dislocations. They evaluated 74 nonoperatively and 132 operatively treated knee dislocations and found significantly improved Lysholm scores in the surgically managed cohort as compared to the cohort treated nonoperatively [39]. Several other studies have corroborated these findings by comparing return to sport following acute knee dislocation and demonstrated higher success rates in those undergoing surgical reconstruction [45, 46].

14.12 Nonoperative Treatment

Despite the emerging clinical evidence that favors operative rather than nonoperative definitive care, there are some instances in which the treating clinician should opt for nonoperative management. Polytraumatized or significantly injured patients with multiorgan system injuries should not be indicated for surgery until they are able to participate in postoperative rehabilitation. Patients with open injuries and inadequate soft tissue coverage in which there are concerns for wound healing should not be indicated for surgical reconstruction. The low functional demand and morbidly obese patient populations will likely have better outcomes with nonoperative rather than operative treatment. Lastly, patients who wish to pursue nonsurgical treatment should be counseled on the pros and cons of both surgical and nonsurgical care and ultimately have their wishes granted if they choose nonoperative management.

14.13 Surgical Treatment

The objective of definitive surgical management following an acute knee dislocation is to provide a stable joint and ideally return the patient to his or her preoperative activity level. While the objective is clearly defined, there is considerable debate concerning several surgical factors, including timing of surgery, surgical approach, ligamentous repair versus reconstruction, and technique of reconstruction.

14.13.1 Timing of Surgery

The timing of surgery can be broadly classified as early (within the first 2–3 weeks following injury) or delayed (greater than 3 weeks from the time of injury). A third broad classification is a staged approach in which the medial and lateral structures are repaired or reconstructed with or without PCL reconstruction in the early window followed by delayed ACL reconstruction if deemed necessary. Although not universally implemented, the staged approach is still in practice and has been advocated by a number of authors [11, 47]. Currently, most knee surgeons advocate early surgical intervention, and this approach is widely supported by the literature [41, 44, 48, 49]. Harner reported on the subjective and objective outcomes of 31 knee dislocations, 19 of which underwent acute reconstructions [41]. Their cohort of acutely treated patients reported higher subjective scores and had increased stability compared to the delayed cohort. Conversely, authors have also reported favorable outcomes utilizing a delayed approach to ligamentous reconstruction [50–54]. Mook and colleagues performed a systematic review of multiligamentous knee injuries treated with early, late, or staged reconstructions [50]. Their analysis suggested that delayed reconstruction had the advantage of lower rates of postoperative stiffness while performing comparable to early and staged procedures in terms of knee stability. Ultimately, the decision to proceed with acute or delayed reconstruction should be based on patient-specific factors and the surgeon's comfort level with the various surgical techniques. Lastly, regardless of the decision to operate in the early or delayed postoperative window, the surgeon should be aware that arthroscopic reconstruction in the presence of a disrupted capsule may cause fluid extravasation and result in compartment syndrome. Although this concern is greater in the immediate post-injury phase, all surgeons should be aware of this potential complication and allow 1–2 weeks of post-injury healing prior to any arthroscopic procedure.

14.13.2 Surgical Technique

A wide variety of surgical techniques have been described for the treatment of acute knee dislocations. Successful surgical intervention first requires the treating surgeon to accurately and completely identify all injuries, including those to ligaments, bone, menisci, cartilage, and adjacent soft tissues. Second, regardless of technique, the primary ligamentous restraints must be repaired or reconstructed in an anatomic and isometric fashion. A detailed discussion of all the potential techniques for the surgical care of acute knee dislocations is outside the scope of this chapter; however, a brief description of our preferred ligament reconstruction surgical techniques will follow.

Once the patient is in the operating room, the first step to a successful knee reconstruction is an examination under anesthesia (EUA). A thorough EUA takes advantage of full muscle relaxation and allows the surgeon to completely delineate the extent of the ligamentous injury. The previously described ligamentous examination is repeated, including Lachman, pivot-shift, anterior and posterior drawers, varus and valgus stress testing, and medial and lateral rotational testing. If there is any uncertainty regarding the extent of ligamentous injury after the MRI and EUA, a diagnostic arthroscopy can be performed prior to autologous graft harvest or open surgical treatment of collateral, PLC, or PMC structures. An initial arthroscopy is also beneficial for evaluation of the menisci, chondral surfaces, and joint capsule (Fig. 14.4a).

14.13.3 Cruciate Ligament Reconstruction

Arthroscopic reconstruction of both cruciates, ACL and PCL, requires anatomic graft placement at the footprints of the native ligaments. Several techniques and graft types are acceptable, and our preferences are for arthroscopic anteromedial single-bundle ACL reconstruction and arthroscopic double-bundle tibial inlay PCL reconstruction [55, 56]. With regard to graft type, for more severe ligamentous injuries that include three or four ligaments and adjacent soft tissue trauma, we prefer to limit the additional donor-site morbidity from graft harvest associated with autograft ligament reconstruction. In this case, we prefer tibialis anterior allograft for

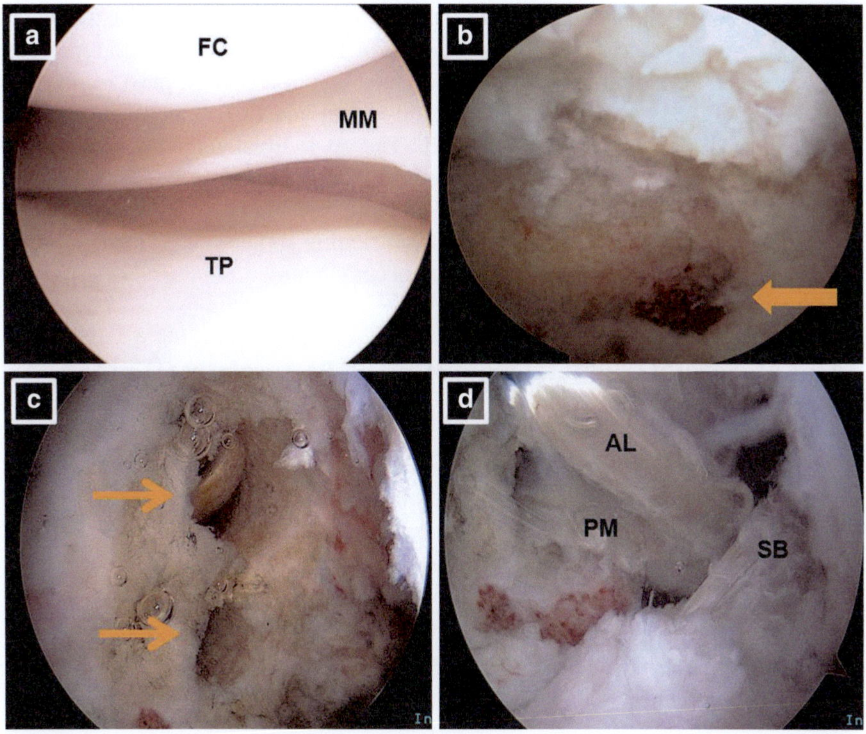

Fig. 14.4 (**a**) Diagnostic arthroscopy image assessing the articular cartilage (femoral condyle (*FC*) and tibial plateau (*TP*)) and menisci (medial meniscus (*MM*)). (**b**) Arthroscopic image with arrow denoting the drilled tibial socket of the posterior cruciate ligament (*PCL*). (**c**) Arthroscopic image with *two arrows* denoting the double-bundle PCL femoral tunnels. (**d**) Arthroscopic image of bicruciate ligament reconstruction with soft tissue grafts in place. The double-bundle PCL reconstruction is labeled by bundle: anterolateral (*AL*) and posteromedial (*PM*). The single-bundle (*SB*) anterior cruciate ligament reconstruction is also shown

ACL reconstruction and Achilles tendon allograft for a bifid double-bundle PCL reconstruction. Hamstring allograft is an acceptable alternative for ACL reconstruction. The potential drawbacks of allograft usage—disease transmission, increased cost, and delayed re-ligamentization—are outweighed by the decrease in operative time, lack of donor-site morbidity, decrease in skin incisions, and reduction in postoperative pain and stiffness [57, 58]. If the decision is made to utilize autograft, preference is given to the ACL. In isolated ACL reconstructions, studies suggest that autograft outperforms allograft in the young, active patient population, and this philosophy is extrapolated to our multiligament reconstructions [59]. The autograft of choice is bone-patellar tendon-bone; however, hamstring and quadriceps tendons are also viable options. If both ACL and PCL are to be reconstructed with autograft, our preference is to use ipsilateral quadriceps tendon for the double-bundle PCL graft. However, rarely do we perform autograft bicruciate ligament reconstruction secondary to the aforementioned drawbacks and potential complications. Bicruciate ligament reconstructions require precise tunnel locations, and to increase the likelihood of this occurrence, the tunnels should be drilled in a consistent and reproducible order. The PCL tibial inlay socket is created first as this is the most technically challenging (Fig. 14.4b). The ACL femoral tunnel and PCL femoral tunnels are drilled after the PCL tibial inlay socket. The ACL tibial tunnel is drilled last (Fig. 14.4c). The grafts are then passed, and the PCL graft is tensioned with the knee in 90° of flexion. The ACL graft is subsequently tensioned with the knee in full extension (Fig. 14.4d) [60]. Of note, graft tensioning should not be finalized until collateral ligament repair or reconstruction is complete.

14.13.4 Lateral Collateral Ligament and Posterolateral Corner Reconstruction

If the MRI findings (LCL attenuation) and EUA (varus opening at 30° without rotational instability) are consistent with an isolated LCL injury, then an LCL reconstruction is indicated. A lateral approach between ITB and biceps femoris is taken to expose the native LCL from origin to insertion (Fig. 14.5a). Our preferred technique is to utilize an Achilles tendon allograft. The allograft bone plug is seated in the proximal fibula and the soft tissue end whipstitched and docked in a femoral bone tunnel proximally. The reconstruction is tensioned in 30° of knee flexion with a valgus force applied. The native LCL is then imbricated or oversewn into the reconstruction.

Injuries to the PLC complex affecting more than the LCL are again addressed through a lateral approach to the knee (Fig. 14.5a). A select group of PLC injuries, in which a distal soft tissue or bony avulsion has occurred, may be amenable to early repair (less than 2 weeks). The repair may be carried out with suture anchors or a screw and washer to reattach the LCL and biceps femoris to their distal attachment sites (Fig. 14.5b). Outside the 2-week window or if mid-substance attenuation exists, scarring and retraction make repair a less reliable option and we advocate surgical reconstruction. The main constituents of the PLC (LCL, popliteofibular ligament, and popliteus tendon) can be reconstructed with one Achilles tendon allograft [61]. The bone plug is secured with an interference screw at the popliteus tendon insertion. The Achilles tendon is then split into two 6–7-mm limbs starting 1–2 cm from the bone plug. The first limb is passed through a fibular bone tunnel (posterosuperior to anteroinferior) and secured with an interference screw to reconstitute the popliteofibular ligament. The residual graft material of this limb is then used to create the LCL. This is accomplished by fixing the graft at the fibular insertion of the LCL with a suture anchor and bringing the graft limb proximally to be passed through a bone tunnel at the anatomic femoral origin of the LCL. The second graft limb is used to recreate the popliteus and is thus passed through a tibial bone tunnel from posterior to anterior at the musculotendinous junction (Fig. 14.5c, d). The graft is tensioned in 30° of knee flexion with internal tibial rotation.

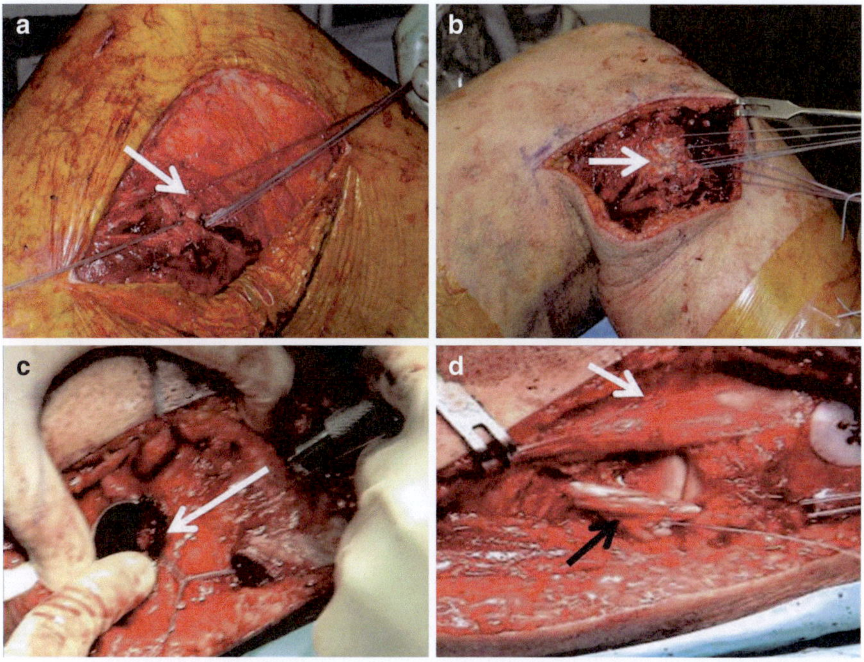

Fig. 14.5 (**a**) Photograph of the lateral approach to the knee with iliotibial band split and biceps femoris and lateral collateral ligament (LCL) exposed (*white arrow*) and tagged with suture. (**b**) Photograph with arrow demonstrating the LCL and posterolateral corner (PLC) elevated in a sleeve and tagged for acute repair. (**c**) Photograph of the drill angle (*white arrow*) and position of the anteroposterior tibial tunnel for recreation of the popliteus component of the PLC. (**d**) PLC reconstruction with popliteofibular ligament graft (*black arrow*), popliteus tendon graft, and LCL graft (*white arrow*) reconstructions

14.13.5 Medial Collateral Ligament and Posterior Medial Corner Repair and Reconstruction

Medial-sided injuries are surgically treated less frequently than lateral-sided injuries. Most cases of MCL and PMC patholaxity in the setting of multiligamentous knee injuries are treated nonoperatively with bracing and protected weight bearing followed by delayed cruciate reconstruction [10]. If, at the time of cruciate reconstruction, there is continued laxity suggestive of a nonhealing grade III injury to the MCL or combined MCL-PMC injury, then MCL-PMC repair or reconstruction is undertaken. A standard medial longitudinal incision centered over the posterior third of the medial femoral condyle is utilized to identify the native MCL. Proximal and distal avulsion injuries are whipstitched and reapproximated to the native attachment site with either suture anchors or a screw and soft tissue washer [33]. The knee is placed in 30° of flexion for appropriate MCL tensioning. The posterior oblique ligament (POL) is reapproximated to the posterior edge of the

MCL with nonabsorbable suture. In cases of mid-substance MCL tears, the opposing ends of the MCL are whipstitched and reapproximated. The medial capsule may also be incorporated into the MCL repair. Likewise, the POL is imbricated into the MCL in a pants-over-vest pattern [33, 62]. Again, the knee should be placed in 30° of flexion during this procedure. Rarely will residual laxity be present with valgus stress testing; however, if valgus patholaxity persists, a soft tissue allograft can be used to supplement the native MCL. The soft tissue allograft should be secured to the native MCL origin and insertion sites with interference screws in bone tunnels or suture anchors.

Often the medial meniscus will need repair, and this can be accomplished with all-inside, inside-out, or hybrid technique. The meniscal attachments to the deep MCL and the posteromedial capsule should also be reapproximated to restore appropriate dissipation of hoop stress through the meniscus [33, 63]. This repair and reapproximation should be completed prior to addressing the MCL and POL.

14.14 Rehabilitation

The overall objective of rehabilitation is to protect the reconstructed or repaired knee in the early postoperative period and then gradually increase motion and strength of the knee over time. There are a number of rehabilitation protocols in the literature with demonstrated good to excellent results [64–66]. In the early postoperative period (33 weeks), the patient is placed in a long-leg splint or hinged knee brace locked in extension. During this time they should remain non-weight-bearing. The non-weight-bearing period may be extended to 6 weeks if fracture fixation, chondroplasty, or meniscal repair is undertaken. Additionally, the non-weight-bearing period may be lengthened due to patient compliance and muscle function. During this time period isometric quadriceps exercises are permitted and electrical muscle stimulation is used to enhance quadriceps recruitment [67]. Early passive motion is initiated between the third and sixth postoperative weeks with a goal of full extension and 90° of passive knee flexion at week six. Achievement of early passive motion goals is often assisted by the use of a continuous passive motion machine for 1 h a day.

The second phase of rehabilitation begins with partial weight bearing at 25 % of body weight. This phase characteristically begins at the sixth postoperative week but again depends on the extent of injury and the patient's ability to demonstrate neuromuscular control of the operative extremity. Once partial weight bearing is initiated, the weight-bearing status is increased by 25 % per week until full weight bearing is resumed. The weight-bearing exercise has a beneficial effect on rebuilding atrophic muscle while providing mechanical stimulus to encourage tendon-to-bone healing in the ligament reconstructions. In a similar fashion, knee flexion is advanced weekly with the goal of 120° of flexion by the 12th postoperative week. All range-of-motion progress is made while wearing a hinged kneed brace, which provides varus/valgus stability to the healing knee. The stationary bike is also incorporated into this phase of the rehabilitation to promote increases in range of motion and quadriceps strength.

From the third to the sixth postoperative month, weight-bearing exercises are advanced and low-resistance quadriceps exercises are introduced. Resisted hamstring exercises are introduced after resisted quadriceps exercises due to the strain hamstring exercises can place on the healing PCL reconstruction. The focus is on closed-chain exercises, as open-chain exercises should be avoided. Proprioception and balance exercises are also introduced during this phase of rehabilitation. Once the quadriceps strength is greater than or equal to 70 % of the contralateral leg, activities may be gradually increased. Jogging and non-cutting activity can begin between the 6th and 9th postoperative months. Emphasis is placed on smooth and slow closed-chain endurance exercise, and jumping rope may be introduced. Plyometrics and cutting activity (sporting activity) are generally resumed between the 9th and 12th postoperative months. If pool workouts and swimming are to be used during the later phases of rehabilitation, it is important to restrict patients from frog kicking or breaststroke until rehabilitation is complete. We use isokinetic strength equivalent to 90 % of the contralateral limb and the single-leg hop test equivalent to 90 % of the contralateral limb as strict criteria prior to returning to sport. Additionally, the patient must be without pain, swelling, and significant laxity to be released to all activity.

14.15 Conclusion

Acute knee dislocations are uncommon yet serious injuries with significant potential for associated neurovascular complications. A high index of suspicion, appropriate clinical examination, and proper diagnostic modalities are paramount to the identification of the complete injury pattern. Vascular and open injuries should be addressed immediately. Osseous injuries should be addressed with open reduction and internal fixation prior to ligamentous reconstruction. The decision to proceed with multiligament reconstruction is multifactorial, and both patient-specific and surgeon factors should impact when and how the multiligamentous knee is repaired or reconstructed. The objectives of treatment and rehabilitation of the acute knee dislocation are to provide a stable, functional knee and ideally to return the patient to an acceptable activity level.

References

1. Brautigan B, Johnson DL (2000) The epidemiology of knee dislocations. Clin Sports Med 19(3):387–397
2. Levy BA, Marx RG (2009) Outcome after knee dislocation. Knee Surg Sports Traumatol Arthrosc 17(9):1011–1012
3. Seroyer ST, Musahl V, Harner CD (2008) Management of the acute knee dislocation: the Pittsburgh experience. Injury 39(7):710–718
4. Shelbourne KD, Pritchard J, Rettig AC, McCarroll JR, Vanmeter CD (1992) Knee dislocations with intact PCL. Orthop Rev 21(5):607–608, 610–601
5. Wascher DC, Dvirnak PC, DeCoster TA (1997) Knee dislocation: initial assessment and implications for treatment. J Orthop Trauma 11(7):525–529

6. Bratt HD, Newman AP (1993) Complete dislocation of the knee without disruption of both cruciate ligaments. J Trauma 34(3):383–389
7. Cooper DE, Speer KP, Wickiewicz TL, Warren RF (1992) Complete knee dislocation without posterior cruciate ligament disruption. A report of four cases and review of the literature. Clin Orthop Relat Res 284:228–233
8. Hoover NW (1961) Injuries of the popliteal artery associated with fractures and dislocations. Surg Clin North Am 41:1099–1112
9. Jones RE, Smith EC, Bone GE (1979) Vascular and orthopedic complications of knee dislocation. Surg Gynecol Obstet 149(4):554–558
10. Klimkiewicz JJ, Petrie RS, Harner CD (2000) Surgical treatment of combined injury to anterior cruciate ligament, posterior cruciate ligament, and medial structures. Clin Sports Med 19(3):479–492, vii
11. Yeh WL, Tu YK, Su JY, Hsu RW (1999) Knee dislocation: treatment of high-velocity knee dislocation. J Trauma 46(4):693–701
12. Kennedy JC (1963) Complete dislocation of the knee joint. J Bone Joint Surg Am 45:889–904
13. Levitsky KA, Berger A, Nicholas GG, Vernick CG, Wilber JH, Scagliotti CJ (1988) Bilateral open dislocation of the knee joint. A case report. J Bone Joint Surg Am 70(9):1407–1409
14. Shelbourne KD, Porter DA, Clingman JA, McCarroll JR, Rettig AC (1991) Low-velocity knee dislocation. Orthop Rev 20(11):995–1004
15. Pace A, Fergusson C (2004) Spontaneous non-traumatic dislocation of the knee. Acta Orthop Belg 70(5):498–501
16. Shetty RR, Mostofi SB, Housden PL (2005) Knee dislocation of a morbidly obese patient: a case report. J Orthop Surg (Hong Kong) 13(1):76–78
17. Green NE, Allen BL (1977) Vascular injuries associated with dislocation of the knee. J Bone Joint Surg Am 59(2):236–239
18. Schenck RC Jr (1994) The dislocated knee. Instr Course Lect 43:127–136
19. Collicott PE (1992) Advanced Trauma Life Support (ATLS): past, present, future–16th Stone Lecture, American Trauma Society. J Trauma 33(5):749–753
20. McCoy GF, Hannon DG, Barr RJ, Templeton J (1987) Vascular injury associated with low-velocity dislocations of the knee. J Bone Joint Surg Br 69(2):285–287
21. Meyers MH, Harvey JP Jr (1971) Traumatic dislocation of the knee joint. A study of eighteen cases. J Bone Joint Surg Am 53(1):16–29
22. Peck JJ, Eastman AB, Bergan JJ, Sedwitz MM, Hoyt DB, McReynolds DG (1990) Popliteal vascular trauma. A community experience. Arch Surg 125(10):1339–1343; discussion 1343–1344
23. Mills WJ, Barei DP, McNair P (2004) The value of the ankle-brachial index for diagnosing arterial injury after knee dislocation: a prospective study. J Trauma 56(6):1261–1265
24. Marin EL, Bifulco SS, Fast A (1990) Obesity. A risk factor for knee dislocation. Am J Phys Med Rehabil 69(3):132–134
25. Robertson A, Nutton RW, Keating JF (2006) Dislocation of the knee. J Bone Joint Surg Br 88(6):706–711
26. Monahan TJ (2001) Management of acute and chronic nerve injuries in the multiple ligament injured knee. Sports Med Arthrosc Rev 9(3):227–238
27. Jonsson T, Althoff B, Peterson L, Renstrom P (1982) Clinical diagnosis of ruptures of the anterior cruciate ligament: a comparative study of the Lachman test and the anterior drawer sign. Am J Sports Med 10(2):100–102
28. Sekiya JK, Whiddon DR, Zehms CT, Miller MD (2008) A clinically relevant assessment of posterior cruciate ligament and posterolateral corner injuries. Evaluation of isolated and combined deficiency. J Bone Joint Surg Am 90(8):1621–1627
29. Borden PS, Johnson DL (2001) Initial assessment of the acute and chronic multiple ligament-injured knee. Sports Med Arthrosc Rev 9(3):178–184
30. Norwood LA Jr, Hughston JC (1980) Combined anterolateral-anteromedial rotatory instability of the knee. Clin Orthop Relat Res 147:62–67

31. Hughston JC, Barrett GR (1983) Acute anteromedial rotatory instability. Long-term results of surgical repair. J Bone Joint Surg Am 65(2):145–153
32. Ritchie JR, Bergfeld JA, Kambic H, Manning T (1998) Isolated sectioning of the medial and posteromedial capsular ligaments in the posterior cruciate ligament-deficient knee. Influence on posterior tibial translation. Am J Sports Med 26(3):389–394
33. Tibor LM, Marchant MH Jr, Taylor DC, Hardaker WT Jr, Garrett WE Jr, Sekiya JK (2011) Management of medial-sided knee injuries, part 2: posteromedial corner. Am J Sports Med 39(6):1332–1340
34. Lunden JB, Bzdusek PJ, Monson JK, Malcomson KW, Laprade RF (2010) Current concepts in the recognition and treatment of posterolateral corner injuries of the knee. J Orthop Sports Phys Ther 40(8):502–516
35. Griffith CJ, Wijdicks CA, LaPrade RF, Armitage BM, Johansen S, Engebretsen L (2009) Force measurements on the posterior oblique ligament and superficial medial collateral ligament proximal and distal divisions to applied loads. Am J Sports Med 37(1):140–148
36. Garavaglia G, Lubbeke A, Dubois-Ferriere V, Suva D, Fritschy D, Menetrey J (2007) Accuracy of stress radiography techniques in grading isolated and combined posterior knee injuries: a cadaveric study. Am J Sports Med 35(12):2051–2056
37. Bui KL, Ilaslan H, Parker RD, Sundaram M (2008) Knee dislocations: a magnetic resonance imaging study correlated with clinical and operative findings. Skeletal Radiol 37(7):653–661
38. Howells NR, Brunton LR, Robinson J, Porteus AJ, Eldridge JD, Murray JR (2011) Acute knee dislocation: an evidence based approach to the management of the multiligament injured knee. Injury 42(11):1198–1204
39. Dedmond BT, Almekinders LC (2001) Operative versus nonoperative treatment of knee dislocations: a meta-analysis. Am J Knee Surg 14(1):33–38
40. Fanelli GC, Orcutt DR, Edson CJ (2005) The multiple-ligament injured knee: evaluation, treatment, and results. Arthroscopy 21(4):471–486
41. Harner CD, Waltrip RL, Bennett CH, Francis KA, Cole B, Irrgang JJ (2004) Surgical management of knee dislocations. J Bone Joint Surg Am 86-A(2):262–273
42. Sisto DJ, Warren RF (1985) Complete knee dislocation. A follow-up study of operative treatment. Clin Orthop Relat Res 198:94–101
43. Almekinders LC, Dedmond BT (2000) Outcomes of the operatively treated knee dislocation. Clin Sports Med 19(3):503–518
44. Levy BA, Dajani KA, Whelan DB et al (2009) Decision making in the multiligament-injured knee: an evidence-based systematic review. Arthroscopy 25(4):430–438
45. Richter M, Bosch U, Wippermann B, Hofmann A, Krettek C (2002) Comparison of surgical repair or reconstruction of the cruciate ligaments versus nonsurgical treatment in patients with traumatic knee dislocations. Am J Sports Med 30(5):718–727
46. Wong CH, Tan JL, Chang HC, Khin LW, Low CO (2004) Knee dislocations–a retrospective study comparing operative versus closed immobilization treatment outcomes. Knee Surg Sports Traumatol Arthrosc 12(6):540–544
47. Ohkoshi Y, Nagasaki S, Shibata N, Yamamoto K, Hashimoto T, Yamane S (2002) Two-stage reconstruction with autografts for knee dislocations. Clin Orthop Relat Res 398:169–175
48. Liow RY, McNicholas MJ, Keating JF, Nutton RW (2003) Ligament repair and reconstruction in traumatic dislocation of the knee. J Bone Joint Surg Br 85(6):845–851
49. Wascher DC, Schenck RC Jr (2001) Surgical treatment of acute and chronic anterior cruciate ligament/posterior cruciate ligament/lateral sided injuries of the knee. Sports Med Arthrosc Rev 9(3):199–207
50. Mook WR, Miller MD, Diduch DR, Hertel J, Boachie-Adjei Y, Hart JM (2009) Multiple-ligament knee injuries: a systematic review of the timing of operative intervention and postoperative rehabilitation. J Bone Joint Surg Am 91(12):2946–2957
51. Fanelli GC, Edson CJ (2004) Combined posterior cruciate ligament-posterolateral reconstructions with Achilles tendon allograft and biceps femoris tendon tenodesis: 2- to 10-year follow-up. Arthroscopy 20(4):339–345

52. Fanelli GC, Giannotti BF, Edson CJ (1996) Arthroscopically assisted combined posterior cruciate ligament/posterior lateral complex reconstruction. Arthroscopy 12(5):521–530
53. Karataglis D, Bisbinas I, Green MA, Learmonth DJ (2006) Functional outcome following reconstruction in chronic multiple ligament deficient knees. Knee Surg Sports Traumatol Arthrosc 14(9):843–847
54. Shelbourne KD, Haro MS, Gray T (2007) Knee dislocation with lateral side injury: results of an en masse surgical repair technique of the lateral side. Am J Sports Med 35(7):1105–1116
55. Bedi A, Altchek DW (2009) The "footprint" anterior cruciate ligament technique: an anatomic approach to anterior cruciate ligament reconstruction. Arthroscopy 25(10):1128–1138
56. Kohen RB, Sekiya JK (2009) Single-bundle versus double-bundle posterior cruciate ligament reconstruction. Arthroscopy 25(12):1470–1477
57. Prohaska DJ, Harner CD (2001) Surgical treatment of acute and chronic anterior and posterior cruciate ligament medial side injuries of the knee. Sports Med Arthrosc Rev 9(3):193–198
58. Shapiro MS, Freedman EL (1995) Allograft reconstruction of the anterior and posterior cruciate ligaments after traumatic knee dislocation. Am J Sports Med 23(5):580–587
59. Borchers JR, Pedroza A, Kaeding C (2009) Activity level and graft type as risk factors for anterior cruciate ligament graft failure: a case–control study. Am J Sports Med 37(12):2362–2367
60. Sherman SL, Chalmers PN, Yanke AB et al (2012) Graft tensioning during knee ligament reconstruction: principles and practice. J Am Acad Orthop Surg 20(10):633–645
61. Sekiya JK, Kurtz CA (2005) Posterolateral corner reconstruction of the knee: surgical technique utilizing a bifid Achilles tendon allograft and a double femoral tunnel. Arthroscopy 21(11):1400
62. Hughston JC, Eilers AF (1973) The role of the posterior oblique ligament in repairs of acute medial (collateral) ligament tears of the knee. J Bone Joint Surg Am 55(5):923–940
63. McAllister DR, Miller MD, Sekiya JK, Wojtys EM (2009) Posterior cruciate ligament biomechanics and options for surgical treatment. Instr Course Lect 58:377–388
64. Edson C (2003) Postoperative rehabilitation of the multiple-ligament reconstructed knee. Oper Tech Sports Med 11(4):294–301
65. Edson CJ (2001) Postoperative rehabilitation of the multiligament-reconstructed knee. Sports Med Arthrosc Rev 9(3):247–254
66. Fanelli GC, Edson CJ (2002) Arthroscopically assisted combined anterior and posterior cruciate ligament reconstruction in the multiple ligament injured knee: 2- to 10-year follow-up. Arthroscopy 18(7):703–714
67. Kim KM, Croy T, Hertel J, Saliba S (2010) Effects of neuromuscular electrical stimulation after anterior cruciate ligament reconstruction on quadriceps strength, function, and patient-oriented outcomes: a systematic review. J Orthop Sports Phys Ther 40(7):383–391

Treatment for Chronic Knee Dislocation

15

Pier Paolo Mariani

Complete knee dislocation is a rare but serious injury. Knee dislocation occurs from high-energy mechanism (motor vehicle or industrial trauma) or from low-energy trauma (sports activity). Vascular and nerve damage, as well as associated fractures or systemic injuries, particularly in high-energy dislocations, contribute to the challenge of treatment. Chronic dislocation may be the result of (1) a missed low-velocity dislocation, (2) a mismanaged high-energy dislocation, or (3) delayed surgery for conditions that preclude operative treatment. Some surgeons prefer a two-staged surgery: an open repair of all capsular lesions and after at least 3 weeks an arthroscopic reconstruction of both cruciate ligaments. With significant capsular damage that does not allow the safe management of the arthroscopic fluid, an open repair of all capsular lesions can be performed within the first 2 weeks of the initial injury. The arthroscopic reconstruction of both cruciate ligaments [1–7] is then postponed until the capsular repair has healed and satisfactory range of motion is achieved.

15.1 Physical Examination

Physical examination is often misleading, especially when the cruciate ligaments and both the medial and lateral collateral ligaments have been damaged. Establishing the neutral anterior-posterior and medial-lateral neutral position is difficult, and the laxity tests are often confusing, leading to a misdiagnosis of lesions. Usually, the laxity is global, and if the ligaments of one compartment have been torn, the opposite compartment ligaments have been at least stretched. Surgical management must address all aspects of the instability and the reconstruction of a single ligament to address this multiplanar instability will result in persistent instability. In order to determine which ligaments are lax or torn, a fluoroscopic stress examination may be

P.P. Mariani
Department of Movement, Human and Health Sciences, University "Foro Italico – Rome 4", Piazza Lauro de Bosis 15, Rome 00135, Italy
e-mail: pierpaolomariani@uniroma4.it

R. Rossi, F. Margheritini (eds.), *Knee Ligament Injuries*,
DOI 10.1007/978-88-470-5513-1_15, © Springer Verlag Italia 2014

helpful, but we prefer to examine the degree of medial or lateral opening at arthroscopy (see below). Ligamentous stability is assessed by a variety of tests and their descriptions are beyond the aim of this chapter. Among the different methods for quantifying anterior-posterior tibial translation, we prefer the Rolimeter (Aircast, Summit, USA) for passive posterior translation and the GNRB system (Genourob, Laval, France) for anterior translation because their measurements correlate well with the clinical examination [8]. For patients with a history of knee dislocation, neurovascular evaluation is critical. The common peroneal nerve is the most commonly injured nerve, with a reported incidence of 14–25 % [9–11]. Therefore, a thorough neurological examination must be performed to document sensory and motor function, in addition to a complete vascular examination.

15.2 Imaging Studies

Plain radiographs should include (1) anteroposterior and lateral views of both knees, (2) bilateral flexion weight-bearing PA view, and (3) stress radiography for posterior and anterior translation, carried out with one of the different described methods. We do not advise stress radiography for varus or valgus because of frequent bias during exam standardization. If available, imaging studies performed immediately after the injury are useful for defining the type and direction of dislocation. In chronic dislocation, MRI is routinely performed and essential for preoperative planning; in addition to associated injuries to the articular cartilage and menisci, MRI can provide detailed information about which structures have been injured.

15.3 Surgical Techniques

There are two key concepts in the operative management of a multiligament knee injury. First, ligament repair and reconstruction must place the attachments for the ligaments and grafts in the normal anatomical attachment site on the femur and tibia. A nonanatomic placement will not appropriately restore the mechanics of the knee. Second key concept is the need for addressing all damaged structures. Operative techniques must deal with all aspects of the instability, and reconstruction of one or two ligaments cannot address this multiplanar instability with persistent instability and disability for the patient. Therefore, preoperative planning is mandatory. The surgical steps are summarized in Table 15.1.

15.4 Anesthesia

At our center, preoperative nerve (femoral and sciatic) block is the preferred method of pain relief for the first 1 or 2 days after ligament surgery. This procedure is not advocated in the presence of peroneal nerve palsy or disease.

Table 15.1 Summary of ligament reconstruction sequence

Diagnostic arthroscopy and meniscal and cartilage treatment
Medial skin incision
Graft harvesting
ACL tibial tunnel
PCL femoral tunnel
PCL tibial tunnel
ACL femoral tunnel
Medial reconstruction
Lateral skin incision
Lateral reconstruction
PCL graft is tensioned in full extension and then fixed at 80° flexion
ACL graft is tensioned and fixed in near full extension
Medial and lateral fixation
Skin closure

15.5 Graft Selection

Considering the multiple grafts needed for this type of surgery, allografts are a logical and valid option. As allografts have limited availability in our country, we are forced to use autografts in chronic dislocation, even if we have some concern about donor site morbidity when harvesting two or more grafts from the same knee. We usually prefer to harvest the quadriceps tendon-patellar tendon or the bone-patellar tendon-bone from the ipsilateral limb for the PCL reconstruction, the hamstring tendon from the ipsilateral limb for the ACL reconstruction, and the hamstring tendon from the contralateral limb for the medial or lateral reconstruction. These options are interchangeable and largely depend on the anatomic lesions being addressed. When allografts are available, the choice depends largely on the surgeon's preference; their main advantages are to minimize donor site morbidity in an already severely injured knee and to reduce the duration of the operation [1, 12–15].

15.6 Arthroscopy

For acute or chronic dislocation, the patient is positioned supine on the operating room table in the decubitus position with the knee flexed 70–90° and the foot on the table. A simple lateral post without a circumferential leg holder is preferred to control the surgical leg, as this allows more freedom for knee motion and can easily be removed if necessary. A tourniquet is used during all surgeries and standard arthroscopy is performed to verify all intra-articular lesions. Five portals are routinely used: (1) superolateral approach for the outflow, (2) anterolateral portal located just inferior to the distal pole of the patella, (3) parapatellar anteromedial portal located just medial to the patellar tendon, (4) posteromedial portal located adjacent to the posterior aspect of the medial femoral condyle and 3 cm above the joint line, and (5) the posterolateral portal located along the posterior edge of the lateral femoral

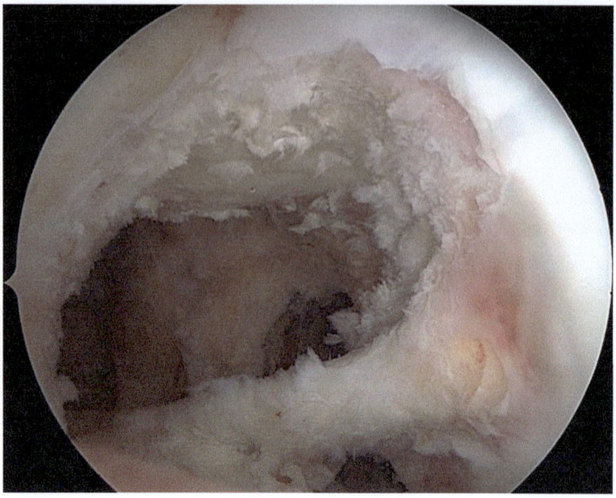

Fig. 15.1 Arthroscopic view of the intercondylar notch, which is "empty" after the removal of scar tissue and preservation of the meniscofemoral ligament

condyle and 1 cm above the joint line. The last portal is performed if necessary or if a transeptal approach will be performed. Diagnostic arthroscopy allows not only an assessment of the status of the articular cartilage and menisci, but is mandatory for planning all of the following surgical steps. The instability pattern is reassessed and compared to the preoperative diagnosis. In detail, disruption of the meniscotibial or meniscofemoral ligament would result in visible elevation of the meniscus from its attachment site on the tibia or femur (meniscal rise sign), which is repaired during the open part of the procedure. The presence of capsular scar tissue or redundancy is noticeable. The intercondylar notch is inspected and any scar tissue debrided. Care should be taken to note the attachment sites of the cruciate ligament and to preserve the meniscofemoral ligaments, if present, even though the meniscofemoral ligaments are often torn or absent in chronic dislocation (Fig. 15.1). The popliteus tendon can easily be visualized and its tension and femoral attachment carefully inspected [16]. Any abnormal opening of the medial or lateral compartment greater than 1 cm, as determined by the "gap test" [17], with varus/valgus stress at 30° is indicative of an injury (Grade III) to the collateral ligament on that side [18].

15.7 Skin Incision

The choice of surgical incision is based on the pattern of ligamentous injuries, with the most common injury being to the ACL, PCL, and MCL or LCL. With the knee in 90° flexion, a curved medial skin incision is made beginning midway between the tibial tubercle and the medial collateral ligament and extending proximally over the medial femoral condyle. This approach allows us to harvest the grafts, create tibial tunnels for ACL and PCL and the femoral tunnel for PCL, and perform MCL and POL reconstructions. At the end of the ACL/PCL arthroscopic reconstruction, if necessary, a lateral hockey stick incision can be made parallel to the posterior edge of the ITT. The incision originates distally just proximal to Gerdy's tubercle and extends proximally to the lateral intermuscular septum. Two or three fascial incisions [19] are made to visualize: (1) the LCL attachment site at the fibula and/or epicondyle, (2) the popliteus tendon and PFL, (3) the biceps tendon, and (4) the peroneal nerve. Neurolysis of the peroneal nerve is routinely performed that is protected throughout the procedure. If the patient has peroneal nerve palsy, we will locate the nerve at this point in the case and decompress it if it is in continuity [10]. In the case of a nerve tear with interruption, we would consider a subsequent surgery for nerve repair and grafting because the rehabilitative protocol for the nerve repair requires a longer period of immobilization.

15.7.1 ACL/PCL Reconstruction

Any autograft tissue is harvested first so that an assistant can prepare the graft on the back table while the surgeon continues the arthroscopic procedure. All of the grafts are kept moist until they are ready to be implanted. We perform an arthroscopically assisted ACL and PCL reconstruction using a single bundle and transtibial procedure for both ligaments. The first tunnel to be created is for the ACL using the Howell tibial guide pin (Arthrotek, Warsaw, IN). The pin is left in place and the tunnel drilled later in order to avoid fluid leakage. For the PCL femoral tunnel, we place only the pin without drilling. Right correct placement of this pin is critical. For single-bundle reconstruction of the PCL, the pin should be located at the center of the anterolateral bundle that is vertical (anterior). Reaching this point is easy using an in-out technique, but the tunnel will be angled too much with a risk of a "killer tunnel." Therefore, we prefer an out-in technique, but in order to reach a point as vertical (anterior) as possible, we use an abrader blade to make a small notch in the roof at 12 o'clock, 5 mm posterior to the articular cartilage. In this way, the tip of a commercial drill guide can easily be placed in the correct position. The bullet of the guide pin is inserted below the bulk of the vastus medialis with the knee flexed 90° and midway between the femoral epicondyle and articular cartilage. Attention is then turned to the PCL tibial tunnel. The scope is shifted from the AL to the PL or the PM portal and a motorized shaver is introduced from the contralateral portal. The posterior septum is removed using the technique described by Ahn et al. [20]. In PCL surgery, a transeptal approach reduces the potential risk to neurovascular structures by providing complete visualization of the tibial PCL insertion and a larger work space. The wider field of vision allows for constant visualization of the tibial tunnel preparation and easier intra-articular passage of the graft. Furthermore, this technique reduces the need to use a 70° scope to view the posterior compartments. The insertion site of the PCL stump on the tibia is easily identified and the fibers of the remaining PCL remnant are dissected subperiosteally. After the posterior tibial sulcus is identified, the arm of the drill guide is inserted from the anteromedial portal and placed in the footprint of the PCL over the attachment of the anterolateral bundle, approximately 1.5 cm below the articular surface and in the midline of the tibia (Fig. 15.2). The guide pin is advanced until it is visualized through the posterior portal. If the pin needs to be repositioned, parallel guide

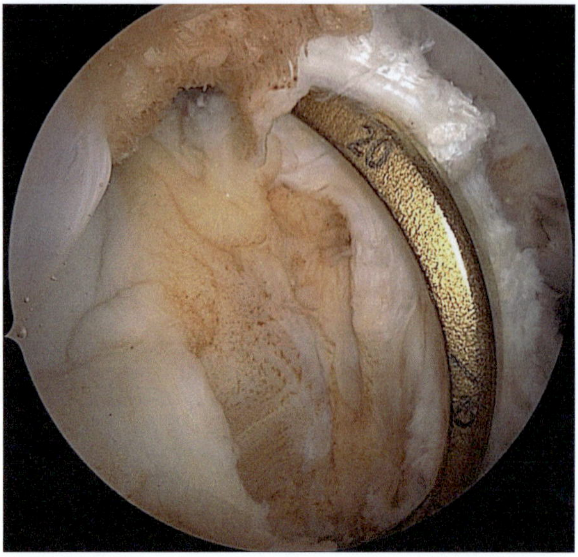

Fig. 15.2 Arthroscopic view from the posteromedial portal of a drill guide placed at the posterior tibial sulcus

pins may be useful. After placing the pin, the tunnel is drilled. Both tibial tunnels are drilled in different directions on the anteromedial surface of the proximal tibia in order to avoid crossing tunnels. Next, the femoral PCL and ACL tunnels are drilled. The edges of all tunnels are smoothed with a rasp prior to passing graft material. The grafts are pulled through the tunnels, the PCL graft first, facilitating intra-articular passage. Every graft-tensioning protocol represents a compromise [21] with a risk of stretching out one or both grafts due to excessive tissue forces, and over time we have changed our protocol. Currently, the ACL/PCL grafts are tensioned after all ligaments have been reconstructed but not yet fixed. The PCL is tensioned first in full extension and then fixed with the knee at 70° flexion, maintaining the tibia in a neutral position and with a "normal" step-off of the medial plateau. Before ACL fixation, we check the restoration of intra-articular points of contact and the restoration of the normal meniscal profile from one of the posterior portals. Then, the ACL is tensioned and fixed with the knee in near full extension. The choice of fixation method depends on the type of graft used.

15.7.2 MCL/POL Reconstruction

Anatomical restoration will proceed from deeper to superficial structures and from posterior to anterior. The deepest layer consists of the meniscotibial and meniscofemoral ligaments. If they are lax at the time of diagnostic arthroscopy, they are re-tensioned with suture anchors with the knee in full extension. The superficial MCL is repaired with a semitendinosus graft, if available [22]. The tendon is left attached distally and a locking suture placed in the end of the graft to facilitate passage under the superficial layer. Anatomical attachment of the MCL on the femur is identified and the isometry of the selected point tested. When the proper femoral position is

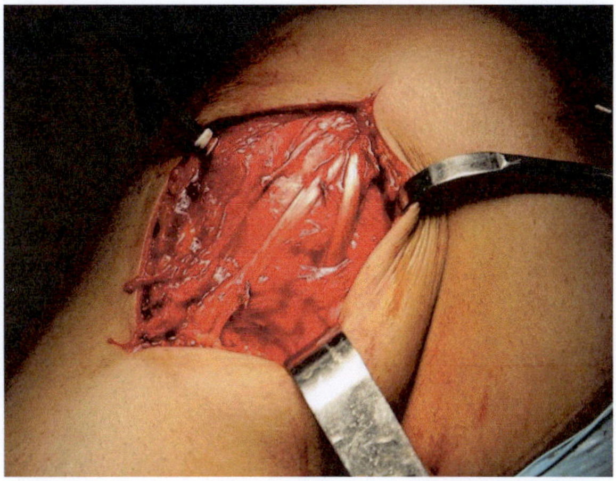

Fig. 15.3 Reconstruction of the superficial medial collateral ligament and the POL using the semitendinosus tendon

found, an eyelet-passing pin is drilled transversely across the femur, and a half-tunnel 25–30 mm in length is reamed according to the measured diameter of the double-looped tendon. With a long-looped suture attached to the eyelet, the tendon is passed through the femoral bone tunnel and secured using an interference screw. While inserting the interference screw, the knee should be held in 30° flexion with varus stress. The free portion of the graft is sutured back to the insertion of the semitendinosus using a permanent suture. An alternative [23, 24] is to perform a "double-bundle" technique that re-creates POL function. A tibial tunnel is drilled to the posterior corner of the medial tibial condyle from anterior to posterior and exits 10 mm below the tibial plateau. The free end of the graft is passed from the femoral condyle through the posterior tibial tunnel opening and fixed with an interference screw (Fig. 15.3). A similar technique has been described with allografts [25, 26]. If the native POL tissue is adequate, a vertical incision is made in the posteromedial capsule between the posterior border of the MCL and anterior border of the POL. The femoral or tibial redundancy is eliminated by imbricating the POL to the MCL in a pants-over-vest fashion or reattaching its insertion to the femur or tibia with suture anchors.

15.7.3 LCL/PL Reconstruction

Surgical options when faced with posterolateral injury can be broadly categorized as fibular-based or tibial-based procedures. The fibular-based reconstruction addresses mainly the varus laxity [27, 28] and consists of a fibular tunnel drilled obliquely (anterolateral to posteromedial) through the fibular head, just distal to the LCL insertion. This site on the fibula can easily be identified by entering the bursa between the long head of the biceps and the LCL. With an incision through the IT band over the lateral epicondyle, the LCL origin, slightly proximal and posterior to the lateral epicondyle, can be exposed. Two options are now possible: (1) pull up the graft into a 6–7-mm tunnel (25–30 mm length so that the notch is not violated) with

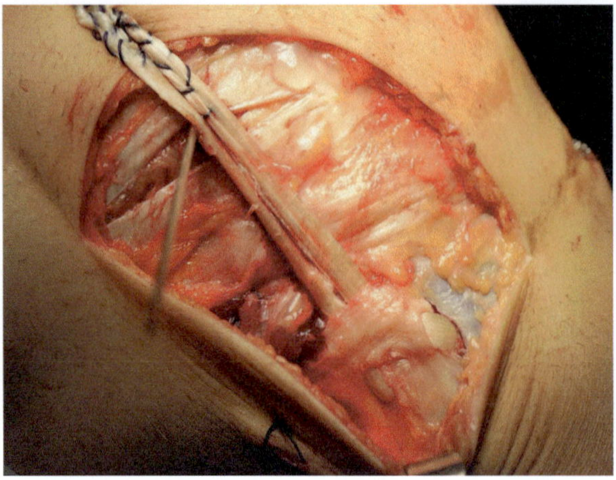

Fig. 15.4 Reconstruction of the lateral collateral ligament using the semitendinosus tendon passed under the long head of the biceps tendon and before passing the ITT. The K-wire is at the femoral site of the native ligament

a passing suture pin and fixing it with an interference screw or (2) secure the graft to the lateral femoral epicondylar region with a screw and to the anatomic insertion site of the LCL with a spiked ligament washer. The tibial-based procedure attempts to re-create the FCL, popliteus, and PFL based on their anatomic origins and insertions to reduce the rotatory laxity [29–35]. The popliteus tendon is reconstructed using a graft strand going from the drill hole opening at the posterolateral tibial condyle to the popliteus tendon insertion point at the femoral condyle. The popliteofibular ligament is reconstructed with a graft strand starting from the posterior aspect of the proximal fibula to the popliteus tendon insertion point at the femoral condyle. Decision-making is based on the preoperative examination, the quality of the tissues at the time of surgery, and the arthroscopic evaluation. Several techniques have been described in the literature with different grafts and fixation methods. Our most commonly used surgical technique for lateral reconstruction is the free graft figure-8 technique using a semitendinosus autograft (Fig. 15.4) and a 2-tailed (fibular head and proximal tibia) technique for the posterolateral reconstruction. When the popliteus tendon looks healthy and the posterolateral capsule is only stretched (i.e., varus test positive and posterolateral drawer and dial tests negative), we use a fibular-based reconstruction. Alternatively, when autografts are not available because they were used for medial reconstruction, a split biceps tendon transfer is used for reconstruction of the FCL [35]. Lax but intact posterolateral structures are tensioned with suture anchors. The PL reconstruction should be tensioned and fixed with the knee in 30° flexion and internal or neutral rotation [36].

15.8 Rehabilitation

At the conclusion of the surgery, the tourniquet is let down and distal pulses confirmed. A dressing is applied and the leg is immobilized in a well-padded, long-leg splint. We use two drains, one intra-articular and one subcutaneous, that are placed to prevent hematoma formation.

Rehabilitation protocols should be individualized according to the specific surgical procedures and the surgeon's preferences. No consensus exists in the literature concerning how slow or fast the rehabilitation must proceed [37, 38], and different protocols have been described [37–42]. Protection of the grafts during the early healing phase must be balanced by the risk of arthrofibrosis, which is reported to be a relative complication after this surgery [5, 43]. In our protocol, the knee should be kept in full extension for 4 or 6 weeks, but we allow range of motion to begin during the first or second week after surgery [39, 40]. If lateral reconstruction is performed, weight bearing is not allowed for the first 6 weeks in order to avoid overstressing these structures. Otherwise, partial weight bearing with crutches is progressed to full weight bearing over the first 4 weeks. After quadriceps control has been reestablished, progressive closed kinetic chain strength training is performed. The patient can return to sports and strenuous labor after the ninth postoperative month, as long as sufficient strength, proprioceptive skills, and motion have returned. Throughout this period, close clinical, functional, and radiographic follow-up is conducted, including MRI studies.

References

1. Delos D, Warren RF, Marx RG (2010) Multiligament knee injuries and their treatment. Oper Tech Sports Med 18:219–226
2. Stannard JP, Brown SL, Farris RC, McGwin G Jr, Volgas DA (2005) The posterolateral corner of the knee: repair versus reconstruction. Am J Sports Med 33:881–888
3. Stannard JP, Bauer KL (2012) Current concepts in knee dislocations: PCL, ACL, and medial sided injuries. J Knee Surg 25:432–456
4. Levy BA, Dajani KA, Morgan JA, Shah JP, Dahm DL, Stuart MJ (2010) Repair versus reconstruction of the fibular collateral ligament and posterolateral corner in the multiligament-injured knee. Am J Sports Med 38:804–809
5. Levy BA, Krych AJ, Shah JP, Morgan JA, Stuart MJ (2010) Staged protocol for initial management of the dislocated knee. Knee Surg Sports Traumatol Arthrosc 18:1630–1637
6. Bin SI, Nam TS (2007) Surgical outcome of 2-stage management of multiple knee ligament injuries after knee dislocation. Arthroscopy 23:1066–1072
7. Ohkoshi Y, Nagasaki S, Shibata N, Yamamoto K, Hashimoto T, Yamane S (2002) Two- stage reconstruction with autografts for knee dislocations. Clin Orthop Relat Res 398:169–175
8. Lefevre N, Bohu Y, Naouri JF, Klouche S, Herman S (2013) Validity of GNRB arthrometer compared to Telos in the assessment of partial anterior cruciate ligament tears. Knee Surg Sports Traumatol Arthrosc. doi:10.1007/s00167-013-2384-4
9. Twaddle BC, Bidwell TA, Chapman JR (2003) Knee dislocations: where are the lesions? A prospective evaluation of surgical findings in 63 cases. J Orthop Trauma 17:198–202
10. Niall DM, Nutton RW, Keating JF (2005) Palsy of the common peroneal nerve after traumatic dislocation of the knee. J Bone Joint Surg Br 2005:664–667
11. Cush G, Irgit K (2011) Drop foot after knee dislocation: evaluation and treatment. Sports Med Arthrosc Rev 19:139–146
12. Fanelli GC, Edson CJ, Reinheimer KN, Garofalo R (2007) Posterior cruciate ligament and posterolateral corner reconstruction. Sports Med Arthrosc 15:168–175
13. Fanelli GC, Tomaszewski DJ (2007) Allograft use in the treatment of the multiple ligament injured knee. Sports Med Arthrosc Rev 15:139–148
14. Fanelli GC, Edson CJ, Beck JD (2010) How I treat the multiple-ligament injured knee. Oper Tech Sports Med 18:198–210
15. Shapiro MS, Freedman EL (1995) Allograft reconstruction of the anterior and posterior cruciate ligaments after traumatic knee dislocation. Am J Sports Med 23:580–587

16. Feng H, Zhang H, Hong L, Wang XS, Zhang J (2009) The "lateral gutter drive-through" sign: an arthroscopic indicator of acute femoral avulsion of the popliteus tendon in knee joints. Arthroscopy 25:1496–1499
17. Noyes FR, Barber-Westin SD, Hewett TE (2000) High tibial osteotomy and ligament reconstruction for varus angulated anterior cruciate ligament-deficient knees. Am J Sports Med 28:282–296
18. LaPrade RF (1997) Arthroscopic evaluation of the lateral compartment of knee with grade 3 posterolateral knee complex injuries. Am J Sports Med 25:596–602
19. Terry GC, LaPrade RF (1996) The posterolateral aspect of the knee. Anatomy and surgical approach. Am J Sports Med 24:732–739
20. Ahn JH, Chung YS, Oh I (2003) Arthroscopic posterior cruciate ligament reconstruction using the posterior trans-septal portal. Arthroscopy 19:101–107
21. Markolf KL, O'Neill G, Jackson SR, McAllister DR (2003) Reconstruction of knees with combined cruciate deficiencies. A biomechanical study. J Bone Joint Surg Am 85:1768–1774
22. Yoshiya S, Kuroda R, Mizuno K, Yamamoto T, Kurosaka M (2005) Medial collateral ligament reconstruction using autogenous hamstring tendons: technique and results in initial cases. Am J Sports Med 33:1380–1385
23. Kim SJ, Lee DH, Kim TE, Choi NH (2008) Concomitant reconstruction of the medial collateral and posterior oblique ligaments for medial instability of the knee. J Bone Joint Surg Br 90:1323–1327
24. Lind M, Jakobsen BW, Lund B, Hansen MS, Abdallah O, Christiansen SE (2009) Anatomical reconstruction of the medial collateral ligament and posteromedial corner of the knee in patients with chronic medial collateral ligament instability. Am J Sports Med 37:1116–1122
25. Borden PS, Kantaras AT, Caborn DNM (2002) Medial collateral ligament reconstruction with allograft using a double bundle technique. Arthroscopy 18:1Y6
26. Fanelli GC, Harris JD (2007) Late medial collateral ligament reconstruction. Tech Knee Surg 6:99–105
27. Larson R (2001) Isometry of lateral collateral and popliteofibular ligaments and techniques for reconstructions using a free semitendinosus tendon. Oper Tech Sports Med 9:84–90
28. Fanelli GC, Larson RV (2002) Practical management of posterolateral instability of the knee. Arthroscopy 18(2 Suppl 1):1–8
29. LaPrade RF, Johansen S, Wentorf FA, Engebretsen L, Esterberg JL, Tso A (2004) An analysis of an anatomical posterolateral knee reconstruction. An in vitro biomechanical study and development of a surgical technique. Arthroscopy 32:1405–1414
30. LaPrade RF, Wentorf F (2002) Diagnosis and treatment of posterolateral knee injuries. Clin Orthop Relat Res 402:110–121
31. LaPrade RF, Ly TV, Wentorf FA, Engebretsen L (2003) The posterolateral attachments of the knee: a qualitative and quantitative morphologic analysis of the fibular collateral ligament, popliteus tendon, popliteofibular ligament, and lateral gastrocnemius tendon. Am J Sports Med 31:854–860
32. Sekiya JK, Kurtz CA (2005) Posterolateral corner reconstruction of the knee: surgical technique utilizing a bifid Achilles tendon allograft and a double femoral tunnel. Arthroscopy 21:1400
33. Jung YB, Jung HJ, Kim SJ et al (2008) Posterolateral corner reconstruction for posterolateral rotatory instability combined with posterior cruciate ligament injuries: comparison between fibular tunnel and tibial tunnel techniques. Knee Surg Sports Traumatol Arthrosc 16:239–248
34. Arciero RA (2005) Anatomic posterolateral corner reconstruction. Arthroscopy 21:1147
35. Zhao J, He Y, Wang J (2006) Anatomical reconstruction of knee posterolateral complex with the tendon of the long head of biceps femoris. Am J Sports Med 34:1615–1622
36. Sigward SM, Markolf KL, Graves BR, Chacko JM, Jackson SR McAllister DR (2007) Reconstruction femoral fixation sites for optimum isometry of posterolateral reconstruction. J Bone Joint Surg Am 89:2359–2368
37. Noyes FR, Barber-Westin SD (1997) Reconstruction of the anterior and posterior cruciate ligaments after knee dislocation: use of early postoperative motion to decrease arthrofibrosis. Am J Sports Med 25:769–778

38. Fanelli GC (2008) Posterior cruciate ligament rehabilitation: how slow should we go? Arthroscopy 24:234–235
39. Stannard JP, Brown SL, Robinson JT, McGwin G Jr, Volgas DA (2005) Reconstruction of the posterolateral corner of the knee. Arthroscopy 21:1051–1059
40. LaPrade RF, Johansen S, Agel J, Risberg MA, Moksnes H, Engebretsen L (2010) Outcomes of an anatomic posterolateral knee reconstruction. J Bone Joint Surg Am 92:16–22
41. Edson CJ (2001) Postoperative rehabilitation of the multiligament-reconstructed knee. Sports Med Arthrosc 9:247–254
42. Fanelli GC, Edson CJ (2002) Arthroscopically assisted combined anterior and posterior cruciate ligament reconstruction in the multiple ligament injured knee: 2- to 10-year follow- up. Arthroscopy 18:703–714
43. Almekinders LC, Dedmond BT (2000) Outcomes of the operatively treated knee dislocation. Clin Sports Med 19:503–518

Postoperative Management: Rehabilitation

16

Ozgur Ahmet Atay, Senol Bekmez, Mehmet Ayvaz, and Gul Baltaci

Multiple ligamentous knee injuries (MLKI) are complex injuries that are often associated with tibiofemoral joint dislocations. Such injuries usually occur with high-energy mechanisms and can be very devastating for the patient. Current approach in treatment is surgical intervention targeting anatomic ligamentous repair or reconstruction. The main goal of treatment is to regain pre-injury activity levels. Rehabilitation is an absolute component of the management to achieve a successful outcome. However, there is limited evidence to build detailed rehabilitation protocols for multiple ligamentous injuries of the knee [1]. Instead, an individualized rehabilitation program with a closed communication between the surgeon, patient, and rehabilitation team should be subjected. Rehabilitation protocols should focus to promote healing, decrease pain and swelling, restore the range of motion (ROM), improve muscle strength and endurance, and enhance proprioception. Rehabilitation must be started as soon as possible in the early postoperative period with concerning the stability of reconstructed and/or repaired soft tissues. Ice and electric stimulation after each exercise session are essential especially in the initial phases of the rehabilitation for pain/inflammation control and quadriceps strengthening. Because of the complexity of the injury, rehabilitative approaches in multiligamentous injuries should be more conservative than those principles valid for isolated ACL ruptures [2].

O.A. Atay (✉) • M. Ayvaz
Department of Orthopaedics and Traumatology,
Hacettepe University Faculty of Medicine, Sihhiye, Ankara 06100, Turkey
e-mail: oaatay@hacettepe.edu.tr; ayvaz@hacettepe.edu.tr

S. Bekmez
Department of Orthopaedics and Traumatology,
Dr. Sami Ulus Training and Research Hospital, Altindag, Ankara 06100, Turkey
e-mail: drbekmez@hotmail.com

G. Baltaci
Department of Physiotherapy and Rehabilitation,
Hacettepe University Faculty of Health Sciences, Sihhiye, Ankara 06100, Turkey
e-mail: ybaltaci@hacettepe.edu.tr

R. Rossi, F. Margheritini (eds.), *Knee Ligament Injuries*,
DOI 10.1007/978-88-470-5513-1_16, © Springer Verlag Italia 2014

Table 16.1 Phases of rehabilitation after MLKI

Week	Goals of the activity
0–6	Pain reduction, rest, icing, elevation
	Muscle reeducation, submaximal quadriceps/hamstring isometrics (pain-free)
	Electrical stimulation with the Swiss ball
	Taping and/or knee bracing in extension
	Scar tissue mobilization
6–10	Single-leg stance balancing and weight shifts
	Gentle quadriceps, hamstrings of motion, and gastrocnemius stretches
	Hip strength and knee stabilization by TheraBand
	Improve knee strength: squatting (30–60–90°)
	Standing electrical muscle stimulation (20 min)
10–24	Restore neuromuscular balance-coordination activities on board
	Quarter squats
	Bicycle, jog, and swim endurance for cardiovascular endurance
	Normal knee strength by using isokinetic system
	Half squats, hamstring curls, lunges, leg press
28–52	Return to sport, sport-specific drills, functional tests, isokinetic evaluation

Current rehabilitation guidelines after ACL/PCL/posterolateral corner and/or medial side reconstructions can be assembled in four consecutive phases lasting approximately 1 year (Table 16.1).

16.1 Phase 1 (0–6 Weeks)

The initial treatment phase includes modalities such as weight-bearing activities to normalize gait, quadriceps strengthening for muscle reeducation, and gentle knee stretches for restoring flexibility. Strict guidelines are to be followed: a home exercise program consisting ice, gastrocnemius and hamstring stretches, heel slides, quadriceps setting, and straight-leg raising (SLR) is emphasized. The appropriate method of exercise in the early phase of soft tissue healing is isometric exercises involving isometric contractions of the quadriceps, hamstrings, and gastrocnemius muscle groups as a cocontraction activity. Modalities as interferential electrical stimulation, cryotherapy, compression, and nonsteroidal anti-inflammatory drugs can be used for decreasing the pain and edema. Electrical stimulation is a supplementary method to regain quadriceps strength [3].

Prolonged immobilization in the early postoperative period is associated with periarticular adhesions and arthrofibrosis that lead to decrease in ROM, destruction of joint cartilage, muscle atrophy, and disuse osteoporosis. Therefore, patellar mobility and quadriceps strengthening/stretching exercises are to be started in the earliest time as pain and effusion would allow. Also to avoid flexion contracture, full passive extension should be gained in the early period with a great precaution not to harm reconstructed tissues.

One of the most important goals to achieve in the initial phase of the rehabilitation is to improve the proprioception and kinesthesia that had been disturbed at the time of the injury. The damaged mechanoreceptors on the injured collateral or cruciate ligaments can never regrow into the grafts. Instead, specific exercises may facilitate the intact mechanoreceptors for compensation. Various exercises that can be used for this purpose are angular joint replication training, end-ROM reproduction training, and perturbation training [4].

In a review of the literature, [5] stated that, continuous passive motion does not provide any substantial advantage following ACL reconstruction, except a possible pain relief. Similarly, Smith and Davies concluded that there was no difference between joint laxity, functional outcomes, postoperative complications, radiological changes, ecchymoses, and muscle atrophy in patients who received continuous passive motion or not [6]. Despite the absence of evidence about any advantages, continuous passive motion may be considered in the immediate postoperative period to decrease postoperative pain.

16.1.1 Early Weight Bearing

The weight bearing must be strictly avoided in the first 4 weeks. Further, as the pain and edema decreases and ROM and neuromuscular control improves, partial weight bearing can be gradually allowed in compliant patients. Besides, a healing time, ranging from 6 to 12 weeks, which is dependent to the type of fixation determines the duration of protection [7]. The timing and amount of weight bearing after reconstruction of isolated ligamentous injuries are well defined. Wright et al. investigated the efficacy of immediate weight bearing versus delayed weight bearing following ACL reconstruction. No deleterious effects of early weight bearing were found regarding stability or function. They suggested that anterior knee pain would decrease with early weight bearing [8]. Following medial collateral ligament (MCL) repairs, non-weight bearing is recommended for the initial 3 weeks with weight bearing as tolerated at 3 weeks; however, effects of early weight bearing are unknown following MCL injury or repair to the MCL [8–10]. Despite that little evidence exists regarding weight-bearing status following posterior cruciate ligament (PCL) injuries, partial weight-bearing status is recommended for 2–4 weeks following PCL surgery to protect the healing structures [11].

In case of multiligamentous reconstructions of the knee joint, no weight bearing for the first week and limited weight bearing for the first 6 weeks is recommended [12]. The effects of early weight bearing following multiligamentous knee surgery are not clear, while early weight bearing following anterior cruciate ligament (ACL) reconstruction is safe without any detrimental effects on stability or function [13].

16.1.2 Knee Bracing

We recommend protecting the reconstructed and repaired tissues with a knee brace locked in extension for 6 weeks postoperatively. After 1 week, controlled non-weight-bearing limited flexion is allowed. Because knee flexion past 100° can increase strain on PCL, knee flexion should be limited at 90° in phase 1 rehabilitation protocols [7].

Despite several studies demonstrated the efficacy of a functional knee brace during early treatment following acute ACL rupture or prophylactic bracing in ACL-deficient knees, there is no evidence to support the routine use of postoperative bracing following ACL reconstruction in systematic reviews [14–17]. However, recent surveys demonstrated that approximately 50–60 % of orthopedic surgeons still use bracing in the early postoperative period following ACL surgery [18].

In the postoperative management of PCL reconstruction, a hinged brace is typically used as the knee is locked in full extension for 2–4 weeks to avoid the effects of gravity and the pulling effect of the hamstrings [19]. However, there is no current evidence indicating that bracing prevents posterior tibial translation [11].

Bracing seems to be beneficial for severe grade II and grade III ruptures of the MCL or following MCL surgery. A long-hinged brace allowing 30–90° of knee motion for the first 3 weeks followed by progressive weaning off the brace starting at week 6 is recommended [9].

16.1.3 Immediate Versus Delayed Mobilization

The current evidence points the benefits of the early mobilization for a successful outcome after ACL and PCL reconstructions. Beynnon et al. summarized five randomized controlled trials on the effects of immediate knee motion as compared to delayed knee motion following ACL reconstruction. The authors concluded that early joint motion after reconstruction of the ACL appears to be beneficial with reduction in pain, lesser adverse changes to the articular cartilage, and helping prevent the formation of scar and capsular contractions that have the potential to limit joint motion [20]. Harner et al. recommend a 2- to 4-week period of immobilization in full extension following a grade III PCL injury to maintain reduction of the tibia and minimize posterior sag to limit forces on the damaged PCL and posterolateral structures. The same recommendations can be applied for following PCL reconstructions [21].

16.2 Phase 2 (6–10 Weeks)

In this phase, the knee brace is unlocked to allow full flexion. The patient is allowed for protective weight bearing to approximately 20 % of body weight with crutches. Furthermore, the weight bearing can be allowed to progress by 20 % each week until full weight bearing is allowed at the postoperative week 10. Any residual flexion contracture can cause extensor mechanism irritation. Although the crutches are discontinued at this point, a multi-instability-specific brace providing anterior-posterior-lateral-medial support is recommended to protect the knee.

In this phase, the goal of knee extension is to obtain and maintain physiologic recurvatum because active neutral extension must be achieved to assume full weight bearing. A gradual increase in passive flexion is allowed to reach the uninvolved side by weeks 8–12. It permits the graft and other soft tissues to adapt the length changes. To not cause early failure on grafts, patient should not be encouraged to attain over 90° of flexion until the end of postoperative week 10. One hundred twenty-five degrees of flexion is adequate even for high-demand activities after week 12.

16.2.1 Neuromuscular Reeducation

Neuromuscular reeducation or neuromuscular (proprioceptive) training has been defined as movement training progressions that facilitate the development of multi-joint neuromuscular engrams that combine joint stabilization, acceleration, deceleration, and kinesthesia through intermittent protocols that progress from low-intensity movements focused in a single plane to multiplanar power training [22]. Cooper et al. investigated the use of proprioceptive and traditional strengthening exercises in individuals with ACL deficiency. Limited improvements were noted in muscle strength, subjective rating, and hop testing following neuromuscular training when compared to traditional strengthening in patients with ACL deficiency [23].

The proprioceptive and kinesthesia exercises progress in a systematic sequence. Partial weight bearing progresses to full weight bearing, double-leg exercises progress to single-leg, single-plane tilt board exercises progress to multi-plane, and open-eye exercises progress to closed eye [24]. Proprioceptive neuromuscular facilitation exercise for hamstrings and quadriceps (Fig. 16.1a, b), progressive resistance training, and balance-coordination exercises for multiligamentous injuries are effective in reducing pain and improving quality of life.

16.2.2 Quadriceps Strengthening

Initial closed chain exercises including wall slides, short-arc squats, multiple direction step-ups, leg press, squat, and lunges should be started in a functional weight-bearing position immediately [25]. Open chain exercises should be avoided especially in case of a patellofemoral disorder [26]. We recommend an exercise progression combining isometric, progressive resistive exercises, balance, kinesthetic ability, coordination, and proprioception in phase 2. Improvement in pain and function can be achieved by using TheraBand in stretching and strengthening exercises (Fig. 16.2). Progressive resistive exercises increase strength, power, and endurance. These exercises consist of three sets of ten repetitions. The first set is 50 % of maximum of ten-repetition weight, the second is 75 %, and the final set is 100 % of the repetition maximum (RM) weight.

Eccentric exercises should be considered to increase muscle strength and functional performance. Gerber et al. evaluated the effectiveness of early progressive eccentric exercise at the 1-year follow-up of ACL reconstruction. Knee extension strength and functional performance improvements were noted in the involved limb in the eccentric group at 1-year follow-up compared to pre-training levels, whereas no improvements were noted in the standard group [27]. Clinicians may also consider the use of eccentric squat program in patients with PCL injury to increase muscle strength and functional performance. MacLean et al. evaluated the efficacy

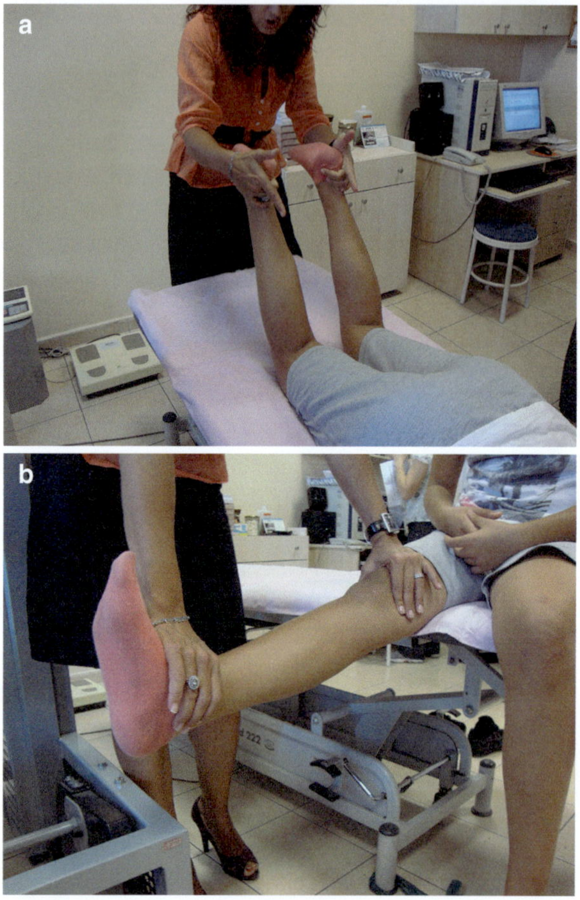

Fig. 16.1 (**a**, **b**) Proprioceptive neuromuscular facilitation techniques for hamstrings and quadriceps

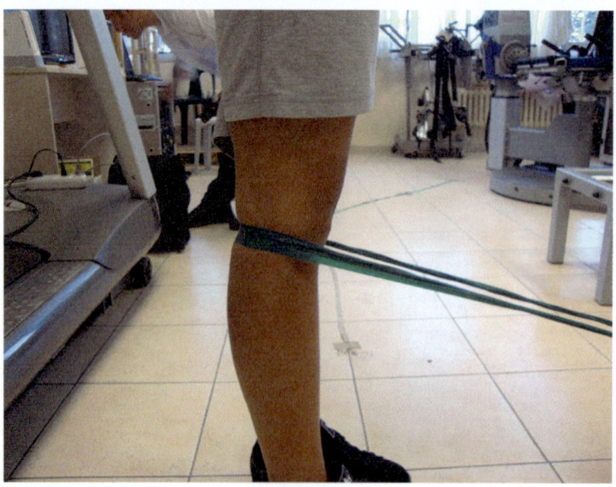

Fig. 16.2 Knee extension quadriceps muscle strengthening by using TheraBand

of a home eccentric exercise program in improving strength, knee function, and symptoms in athletes with PCL injury. Knee functions and symptoms were improved over the 12-week period. The quadriceps in the involved limb showed significantly greater improvement in eccentric torque following eccentric training [28].

16.2.3 Kinesio Taping

Kinesio Taping application, as an increasingly popular method in the rehabilitation and prevention of sports injuries, has been recommended for relief from insidious pain. Kinesio Taping has physiological effects including decreasing pain or abnormal sensation, supporting the movement of muscles, removing congestion of lymphatic fluid or hemorrhages under the skin, and correcting misalignment of joints [29]. After applying Kinesio Taping, the taped area will form convolutions to increase the space between the skin and muscles. Once the skin is lifted, the flow of blood and lymphatic fluid is promoted. We recommend the Kinesio Taping for acute pain and discomfort after surgery (Fig. 16.3a, b).

16.3 Phase 3 (10 Weeks to 6 Months)

The rehabilitation program focuses on improving ROM and increasing quadriceps strength in this phase. The target ROM is approximately 120° in this phase. Closed chain exercises are recommended to enhance proprioception. An advanced modality of quadriceps strengthening is the open kinetic chain exercises that should be initiated only 4 months after the reconstruction. Open chain exercises should proceed with a great caution to avoid inflammation-based anterior knee pain that may alter the progression of rehabilitation protocol. However, resistance should be limited only to the body weight and knee flexion should be limited to 60°, initially. Resistive exercises should include both concentric and eccentric ones to provide functional activities. Dynamic stability, which is required to return various functional activities, is mainly generated by quadriceps, hamstring and gastrocnemius muscle groups [30]. If the patient does not suffer from pain, swelling and discomfort during and after activity, we recommend to add turning, twisting, jumping and running to the rehabilitation program. Furthermore, more functional activities and proprioceptive trainings should be started with the balance board, trampoline jumping, and skipping rope. Once the patient successfully improved in regard to quadriceps strength, straight-line jogging can be permitted at the end of the fifth postoperative month.

16.4 Phase 4 (28–52 Weeks)

Running in nonlinear directions and low-intensity cutting activities can be initiated at months 6 through 9 [31]. Isolated hamstring exercises without resistance and bilateral or single-leg plyometric exercises are also initiated [32]. Consequently,

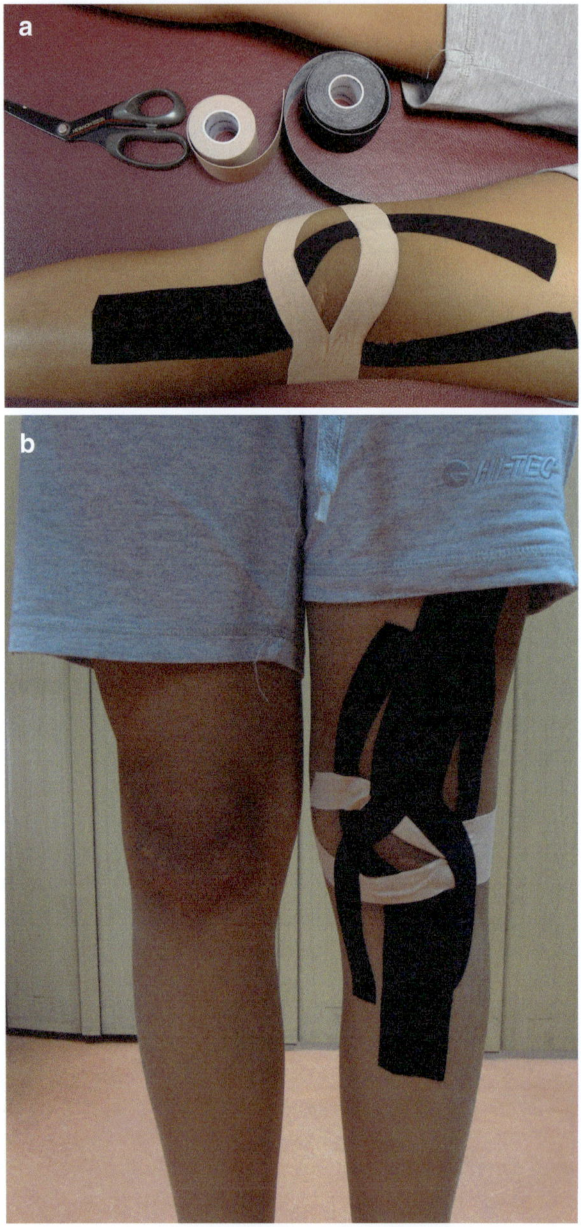

Fig. 16.3 (**a**, **b**) Kinesio Taping application for quadriceps and vastus medialis muscle, mechanical correction for patella, and ligamentous technique

rehabilitation strategies such as perturbation training, plyometrics, advanced agility drills, and ergonomic/sport-specific simulations obtain a controlled clinical environment generating the forces that may create destabilizing forces across the knee [22]. The intended quadriceps strength is at least 90 % of the non-injured side. A 10–15° of terminal flexion loss is common despite aggressive ROM exercises. Any joint soreness and swelling should be monitored carefully for the potential injury risk in efforts to gain full flexion. Completion of the rehabilitation program and return to the manual labor or sportive activity should be regarded at the end of postoperative 9 months. Return to sports should be based on objective measures that assess patient's performance [33]. A functional test algorithm in a step-by-step process should be used to evaluate the patient's progression after rehabilitation program. Prophylactic bracing is a controversial issue but we recommend it until 18 months postoperatively especially during sportive activity.

16.5 Conclusion

In summary, because of the complexity and the rarity of the multiple ligamentous injury patterns of the knee joint, there are no randomized controlled trials regarding ideal rehabilitation guidelines. So, rehabilitation protocols should be individualized to meet the specific needs of the patients. Overall, a systematic and patient-based rehabilitation algorithm can provide a good outcome even in such a devastating condition. If the patient rapidly returns to activity, we perform functional tests such as one-leg hopping and jumping tests indicating neuromuscular control, strength, power, and most importantly knee stability. Repetitions, frequency, and resistance weight of exercises should be modified according to the patient's individual ability. It is important to convince physicians, physical therapists, athletic trainers, coaches, and the athletes themselves to implement active prevention measures into therapy and training programs, thus decreasing the injury and reinjury risks and enhancing athletic performance.

References

1. Irrgang JJ, Fitzgerald GK (2000) Rehabilitation of the multiple-ligament-injured knee. Clin Sports Med 19(3):545–571
2. Edson CJ, Fanelli GC, Beck JD (2011) Rehabilitation after multiple-ligament reconstruction of the knee. Sports Med Arthrosc Rev 19:162–166
3. Snyder-Mackler L, Ladin Z, Schepsis AA et al (1991) Electrical stimulation of the thigh muscles after reconstruction of the anterior cruciate ligament: effects of electrically elicited contraction of the quadriceps femoris and hamstring muscles on gait and on strength of the thigh muscles. J Bone Joint Surg 73A:1025–1036
4. Fitzgerald GK, Axe MJ, Snyder-Mackler L (2000) The efficacy of perturbation training in nonoperative anterior cruciate ligament rehabilitation programs for physically active individuals. Phys Ther 80:128–140
5. Wright RW, Preston E, Fleming B (2008) A systematic review of anterior cruciate ligament reconstruction rehabilitation: part I: continuous passive motion, early weight bearing, postoperative bracing, and home-based rehabilitation. J Knee Surg 21:217–224
6. Smith T, Davies L (2007) The efficacy of continuous passive motion after anterior cruciate ligament reconstruction: a systematic review. PhysTher Sport 8:141–152
7. Lutz GE, Palmitier RA, An KN (1993) Comparison of tibiofemoral joint forces during open and closed kinetic chain exercises. J Bone Joint Surg 75(5):732–739
8. Shelburne KB, Torry MR, Pandy MG (2005) Muscle, ligament, and joint-contact forces at the knee during walking. Med Sci Sports Exerc 37:1948–1956
9. Phisitkul P, James SL, Wolf BR et al (2006) MCL injuries of the knee: current concepts review. Iowa Orthop J 26:77–90

10. Reider B (1996) Medial collateral ligament injuries in athletes. Sports Med 21:147–156
11. Janousek AT, Jones DG, Clatworthy M et al (1999) Posterior cruciate ligament injuries of the knee joint. Sports Med 28:429–441
12. Medvecky MJ, Zazulak BT, Hewett TE (2007) A multidisciplinary approach to the evaluation, reconstruction and rehabilitation of the multi-ligament injured athlete. Sports Med 37:169–187
13. Rihn JA, Groff YJ, Harner CD (2004) The acutely dislocated knee: evaluation and management. J Am Acad Orthop Surg 12:334–346
14. Swirtun LR, Jansson A, Renstrom P (2005) The effects of a functional knee brace during early treatment of patients with a nonoperated acute anterior cruciate ligament tear: a prospective randomized study. Clin J Sport Med 15:299–304
15. Kocher MS, Sterett WI, Briggs KK et al (2003) Effect of functional bracing on subsequent knee injury in ACL-deficient professional skiers. J Knee Surg 16:87–92
16. Birmingham TB, Bryant DM, Giffin JR et al (2008) A randomized controlled trial comparing the effectiveness of functional knee brace and neoprene sleeve use after anterior cruciate ligament reconstruction. Am J Sports Med 36:648–655
17. Wright RW, Fetzer GB (2007) Bracing after ACL reconstruction: a systematic review. Clin Orthop Relat Res 455:162–168
18. Marx RG, Jones EC, Angel M et al (2003) Beliefs and attitudes of members of the American Academy of Orthopaedic Surgeons regarding the treatment of anterior cruciate ligament injury. Arthroscopy 19:762–770
19. Wind WM Jr, Bergfeld JA, Parker RD (2004) Evaluation and treatment of posterior cruciate ligament injuries: revisited. Am J Sports Med 32:1765–1775
20. Beynnon BD, Johnson RJ, Abate JA et al (2005) Treatment of anterior cruciate ligament injuries, part I. Am J Sports Med 33:1579–1602
21. Harner CD, Hoher J (1998) Evaluation and treatment of posterior cruciate ligament injuries. Am J Sports Med 26:471–482
22. Hewett TE, Paterno MV, Myer GD (2002) Strategies for enhancing proprioception and neuromuscular control of the knee. Clin Orthop Relat Res 302:76–94
23. Cooper RL, Taylor NF, Feller JA (2005) A systematic review of the effect of pro- prioceptive and balance exercises on people with an injured or reconstructed anterior cruciate ligament. Res Sports Med 13:163–178
24. Ohkoshi Y, Yasuda K, Kaneda K (1991) Biomechanical analysis of rehabilitation in the standing position. Am J Sports Med 19:605–611
25. Ellenbecker TS, Davies GJ (2001) Closed kinetic chain exercise: a comprehensive guide to multiple joint exercises. Human Kinetics, Champaign
26. Shelbourne KD, Trumper RV (1997) Preventive anterior knee pain after anterior cruciate reconstruction. Am J Sports Med 25:41–47
27. Gerber JP, Marcus RL, Dibble LE et al (2009) Effects of early progressive eccentric exercise on muscle size and function after anterior cruciate ligament reconstruction: a 1-year follow-up study of a randomized clinical trial. Phys Ther 89:51–59
28. MacLean CL, Taunton JE, Clement DB (1999) Eccentric kinetic chain exercise as a conservative means of functionally rehabilitating chronic isolated insufficiency of the posterior cruciate ligament. Clin J Sport Med 9:142–150
29. Williams S, Whatman C, Hume PA (2012) Kinesio taping in treatment and prevention of sports injuries: a meta-analysis of the evidence for its effectiveness. Sports Med 42(2):153–164
30. Ciccotti MG, Kerlan RK, Perry J (1994) An EMG analysis of the knee during functional activities: part II. Am J Sports Med 22:651–658
31. Spencer JD, Hayes KC, Alexander JJ (1984) Knee joint effusion and quadriceps inhibition in man. Arch Phys Med Rehabil 65:171–177
32. Myers GD, Paterno MV, Ford KR (2008) Neuromuscular training techniques to target deficits before return to sports after anterior cruciate ligament reconstruction. J Strength Cond Res 22:987–1014
33. Bjorklund K, Andersson L, Dalen N (2009) Validity and responsiveness of the tests of athletes with knee injuries: the new criterion based functional performance test instrument. Knee Surg Sports Traumatol Arthrosc 17:435–445

MIX
Papier aus verantwortungsvollen Quellen
Paper from responsible sources
FSC® C105338

If you have any concerns about our products,
you can contact us on
ProductSafety@springernature.com

In case Publisher is established outside the EU,
the EU authorized representative is:
Springer Nature Customer Service Center GmbH
Europaplatz 3, 69115 Heidelberg, Germany

Printed by Libri Plureos GmbH
in Hamburg, Germany